Be In Good

Health

Be In Good
Health

Living a Life of Happiness, Wholeness and Wellness!

Cee Cee H. Caldwell-Miller

Brilliance in U Publishing (a division of Brilliance in U Int'l)

The information contained in this book is intended to be educational and from the author's personal experience and not for diagnosis, prescription, or treatment of any health disorder whatsoever. This information should not replace consultation with a competent professional. The author and publisher are in no way liable for any misuse of the material. This publication contains the opinions and ideas of its author. It is intended to provide helpful and informative material on the subject matter covered. It is sold with the understanding that the author and the publisher are not engaged in rendering professional services in the book.

First Printing: October 2008

Second Printing: April 2017

Library of Congress Cataloging-in-Publication Data

Caldwell-Miller, Cee Cee H.

Be In Good Health: Living a Life of Happiness, Wholeness and Wellness/ Cee Cee H. Caldwell-Miller

Includes bibliographical references.

ISBN 9781544771984

1. Health. 2. African American. 3. Wellness 3. Self help 4. Personal Development

Book design: J.T. Miller of iVue Graphics & Media Solutions, Inc.

Back Cover Photograph: Abdur-Rahmaan Ali of Upscale Network NJ

Beloved, I wish above all things that thou mayest prosper and be in health, even as thy soul prospereth.

3 John 1:2

To everyone who has imparted something into my life at one time or another and taught me about accepting myself as God designed me.

To the wellness seekers who are looking to live the life that they were destined to live by being healthy, wealthy and whole.

God's Choicest Blessings!

"Self-Care is the Best Care and it is far Better, than Healthcare!"

The courage to be you

You are unique, with your own special beauty and value to give to life. What a terrible shame it would be if you were to let that beauty be hidden behind your fears.

When you worry that you're not good enough, you allow others to control you, and their domination will soon make you miserable. Or when you fool yourself into thinking you're superior to everyone else, you deny yourself the exquisite joy of offering your own special gifts to life.

It takes courage and faith, effort and initiative to be who you are. And it is so very much worth the effort.

Though no one else can do it for you, you have what it takes to be magnificently successful at being you. From the deepest secrets of your soul to the face you put forward to the world, every bit of you is meant to be the authentic and original person you are.

Listen to that quiet, persistent voice inside that you know is always right. This is your opportunity to fulfill and express the real and lasting joy of being you.

Let the beautiful person inside of you come more fully to life as each moment passes. Let yourself, and the world around you, know the joy and fulfillment that is meant just for you to express.

Ralph Marston

Table of Contents

Spirit

Conclusion

Extras

Foreword Toni Coleman Brown

It has been said that before you can be a better half that you must be a complete whole. Being complete in mind, body and spirit is something that we all strive for and with the information that Cee Cee Caldwell-Miller has expressed in this body of work you will certainly get on the path to becoming whole.

I can remember the time I first met Cee Cee. She was speaking in front of a crowded room of people giving her testimony on why they should become empowered by her network marketing opportunity. When she opened her mouth to speak, I knew that she was filled with a powerful anointing from God. Her spirit glistened with a genuine concern and caring for others and success was not just something that she wished for others to have, it was something that she was also destined for. And right now she is walking in her destiny by sharing with others her ideas and expressions that will help others achieve Wellness in multiple facets of their life.

It is clear from this information that when one aspect of our Wellness Wheel is out of balance, we will not be a complete Whole (individual). It is mandatory for all of us to seek balance, so that our Wellness Wheel is not lop-sided or doesn't look like a balloon, but looks like a perfectly balanced circle. Cee Cee shows us how to look within and make the necessary adjustments to make sure that our Wellness Wheels are equipped to roll us down the roads that represents our own Life's Journey.

In this piece you will discover that your Wellness Wheel has several spokes or facets and it will be up to each individual to design their own wheel (or life). It's like getting rims on a car, we have freedom to adorn them however we choose, but still the wheels must be balanced from their very foundation in order to travel down the road and function properly. So, Cee Cee teaches us to live in balance, from emotional, mental, and financial to physical, social and spiritual health and wellness, she encourages us to be in good health so that we can truly live out God's manifestation for our lives. This is a lesson that all are encouraged to learn.

Toni Coleman Brown
www.qlproductions.com

Preface

I decided to write this book because, it was my belief that when you hear the word health, we so often just think about the physical. Health is much more than how your physical body works, it encompasses so much more. Health involves the physical but it also involves: spiritual, mental, emotional, financial, social, relational, environmental and educational health.

So I wanted to write a book in plain old English, that would encourage people to open themselves up to the possibility of being healthy and whole completely. We were created to be healthy, happy and whole, while living a life of abundance and prosperity. When I speak of abundance and prosperity I am referring to wholeness in mind, body and spirit. There are so many things that cause us to be unhealthy, unproductive and feel unworthy. I have felt all of these things at one point in time but I had to finally make a decision to make a change in my life.

I realized that I deserved a life of happiness, joy and total fulfillment, that's when I decided it, was time to begin my life again. I knew the journey would not be easy, I knew that there would be challenges and setbacks but I was willing to take the chance to see what the future had in store for me. What I began to understand was that in order to become whole and complete, I would have to be willing to fail while trying instead of not trying at all. There is no failure in trying but there is in making excuses for not trying at all. I wanted this project to inspire, encourage and support those who were willing to work to win the prize of a lifetime, which is total wellness. If you are tired of being sick and tired, of not living the life you have always dreamed of or just want to feel better, stronger, happier and more energetic, then this is the book for you. I wrote this book to help you jump-start your new beginning. I have included resources that I believe will help you on your journey to holistic health and wellness. I am not a medical doctor but I am a holistic practitioner/wellness consultant and an experienced wellness seeker. I have tried many of the suggestions outlined in this book, some of which I was successful at and some of which I was not but, I still believe in them all.

My lack of success was not due to the suggestions or methods; it was due to my own lack of discipline and steadfastness. I know you can change your life and become the person that you always knew was there but it will take, time, strength, dedication and support to reach the finish line. It is my aim to equip you with the tools to live your best life from the inside out.

Once you reach your goal in one area of wellness, then move on to the next, remember if some areas are lacking continue to move toward wholeness one step at a time. Every single thing in your life right now -- your job, relationships, money, health, and all that you have intellectually, emotionally and spiritually -- is a reflection of your beliefs. Your belief has the power to attract your deepest desires and so much more than you could have ever imagined. It's all up to you, Get on your mark, get set, and GO!

Acknowledgments

With deepest gratitude I would like to thank everyone who had some hand in the writing of this book.

Firstly, I would like to thank God for putting this project on my heart and trusting me with the information that I believe will be a blessing to the lives of others. If it were not for him, blessing me with the gifts that he has, I would not be writing this book or living today. To God be the glory for the things he has done is doing and will do in my future.

Secondly, I would like to thank the Health and Wellness industry for giving me the opportunity to be a part of such a growing industry and at the same time allowing me to use my ability to help people enrich their lives through my knowledge of better health, wellness and self-care.

Thirdly, I would like to thank all of the powerful women who have impacted my life in one form or another. The women who have inspired me to reach for the top and continue until I reached my goals while striving to live the life that I was purposed and destined to by God.

And finally, I would like to thank everyone who has allowed me to share a part of my life with them and who have been a part of mine at any point in time. I believe that everyone comes into your life for a purpose and a season and I am grateful to all who have blessed my life just by being a part of it, thanks for your unwavering support.

A special thank you goes to Teri Jackson-Carson; from the first time I met Teri through Warm Spirit I felt blessed to learn about the Wellness industry from someone like her. Her love for helping people dance with amazing choreography captured me from the start. Teri caused me to want to learn more about health and wellness and that is why I am able to write this book today. So I bless her and I sincerely thank her for being a great wellness mentor. And I will always remember, "Your Health Is Your Wealth!

Finally, I would like to thank the world for allowing me the pleasure to share my life, my gifts and my love for helping people become the best they can be by helping them on their journey to wholeness and happiness.

Remember, Be in Good Health, and be good to yourself and each other. You Are Worth It!

Cee Cee H. Caldwell-Miller, MA, CPC, ALS

Let Your Journey to Holistic Wellness begin...... Where you start is totally up to you, just make yourself a priority on your own list!

Introduction

Living Life To The Fullest - You must be complete.

Your destiny is not really about what happens to you. It is built and fulfilled by the things that you cause to happen, by what you do with the precious life you have been blessed with. It happens in every moment, with every choice, with every thought and every action. Always remember, you are creating your own unique destiny. If you live your life to the fullest by being rich, not in money but by being whole and complete in every area of my life, you will obtain the prosperity that you were destined for.

As I began to do research for this book, I questioned whether I had the ability to write it or not. And as I pondered the thought, I realized that I didn't have to possess a PhD. in medicine or health to successfully share the knowledge I have gained in the area of health, wellness and self-care. The reason that I feel capable of sharing the information presented, is my own life experiences, choices and training.

My hope is that this book will encourage you to be all that you can be, by working from the inside out to create the YOU that you were meant to be in every area of your life. From your physical health to your moral health, I hope to inspire you to begin the journey or complete the journey that you may have already begun in pursuing complete wholeness in your life.

Whether you are a parent, a teacher, a health professional, or just seeking to better understand yourself and your relationships so you can heal and grow, this book is for you.

Over the years, I have personally struggled with the issues that I will address in this book from physical wellness to emotional wellness and many more. It has been a daily journey for me, toward wholeness and often not an easy one. I have had failures and successes in my life but through my strong faith I have been able to conquer the challenges and push my way through to enjoy the fruit of my labor. I believe that everyone deserves to be whole and happy no matter what experiences they have endured throughout their lifetime. I know that the journey ahead may seem difficult but trust me, it is well worth it and there is definitely light at the end of the tunnel. Let's begin the journey with a look into the area of mental health.

Chapter 1

Mental Health-Sane or Insane

What is Mental Health?

Every aspect of your life, the place you live, the people you live with, your friends and acquaintances, the things you do or don't do, the things you own, your work, even things like pets, music, and color affect how you feel. If you are concerned about your mental health or the quality of your life, you can do many things and make changes in your life that will help you to feel much better.

A calm and undisturbed mind and heart are the life and health of the body, but envy, jealousy, and wrath are like rottenness of the bones. Proverbs 14:30

Having good mental health means that your perceptions and feelings lead you do behave in a normal manner. Mental health is often defined in the negative sense of being free from mental, psychological or emotional disorders. Everyone wants to be mentally healthy, but achieving that goal can be a challenge due to outside forces and your own destructive attitudes.

"Taking care of your mental health to prevent problems should be a major focus. Healing, repair and behavior management are the necessary efforts in restoring mental health once there is a problem. Effectively dealing with psychiatrists, psychologists, therapists and healthcare professionals is also important in recovery." Ron Kurtus (revised 22 September 2002 www.school-for-champions.com}.

It has always been easier to define mental illnesses than to define mental health. In the United States the American Psychiatric Association has traditionally been the organization to define mental disorders (beginning as early as 1917 when it was known as The Association of Medical Superintendents of American Institutions of the Insane). More recently many have recognized that mental health is more than the absence of mental illness. Even though many of us don't suffer from a diagnosable mental disorder, it is clear that some of us are mentally healthier than others. The study of the characteristics that make up mental health has been called "positive psychology." Here are some of the ideas that have been put forward as characteristics of mental health:

• The ability to enjoy life is essential to good mental health.

• The ability to cope with stress and life situations.

• The ability not to take things so seriously.

• The ability to see the good in everything.

• The ability to bounce back from stressful situations.

• The ability to find balance in one's life.

According to Ron Kurtus "just as the body needs good nutrition to sustain its health, so too does the mind need good mental nutrition for its health. This nutrition consists of positive thoughts and feedback from others. Negative thoughts and criticisms from others can be toxic or poisonous and harmful to your mental health." Ron Kurtus (16 January 2006 www.school-for-champions.com}. It is necessary to replace negative self-talk or other negative influences with positive affirmations and positive thinking.

My Story: Over the years, I have had struggles with my mental wellness at times, because of the pressures & stresses of life. It is my belief that everyone could use the assistance of a mental health practitioner. Whether it is a professional counselor, psychologist, minister or friend, find someone to help you sort through your problems, concerns or life situations. It is my belief that we are all one-step from going from sane to insane, if the right situation presented itself. It is important that we develop a strong mental outlook on life and the things around us, so that we may maintain a healthy mental state of mind. I have been on the verge of a total mental breakdown many times, I utilized the tools and coping mechanism that I have learned over the years to bring myself from the brink of a complete mental meltdown. It is important that we are aware of what pushes us to the limit, so that we can counteract the inevitable by knowing how to move pass the mental stresses of life toward a peaceful state of mind. Let's now take a look at our emotional health.

Chapter 2

Emotional Health-Happiness or Sadness

What is Emotional Health?

Optimal state of emotional well-being is essential to achieving overall wellness. Emotional health in this context includes one's ability to appropriately express their emotions, their ability to learn, and their ability to have meaningful social interactions and connections. Maintaining these aspects of emotional health can at times be difficult for all of us especially for university students in particular because of the many adjustments they make while attending university and the high levels of stress many face during the semester, I will address this in a later chapter.

Emotion is an essential aspect of interpersonal communication. The capacity to feel is what makes us human, and what connects us to one another. Emotional intelligence is what helps us to achieve our potential, and to fulfill our hearts' ambitions. So, the more we develop and refine our emotional intelligence the more we can enjoy fulfilling relationships, realize our deepest longings, manage life's conflicts with grace, and create fair, peaceful and sustainable societies. (Grille, Robin. 'Parenting for a Peaceful World." According to Robin Grille, Read 'Parenting for a Peaceful World' and learn:

1.   The five stages of core emotional development in early childhood.

2.   How your early childhood experiences have affected your emotionality, your behavior and your relationships.

3. How to promote your children's emotional intelligence so they can grow to have the most healthy and rewarding relationships with others, and fulfill their potential.

4. Up-to-date research into child development, heredity vs. environment

5. New understandings about the causes of childhood disorders (behavioral and psychological)

6. What leading-edge child-development research implies for early childhood education philosophy

7. New and exciting innovations in the philosophy of early childhood education

8. How child rearing practices have affected societies and international affairs throughout history.

9. How our child rearing choices can be the most powerful agents for positive social change and planetary healing.

Many of the experiences we have in childhood leave a lasting emotional impression, even if we don't consciously recall them. Our emotional health during childhood years has a profound influence on how we relate to each other as adults.

The good news is there is a lot we can do to develop our emotional health as adults. Counseling or psychotherapy can do much to help us develop our emotional health. Conflicts and difficulties can be turned into opportunities for learning, healing, growth and development. Nurturing our emotional health can transform our relationships from unhealthy toxic ones too healthy and fulfilling ones, and in fact, it can change the world.

Since our childhood experiences so strongly influence our emotional health, the way we raise our children is of profound consequence. Which is why you can learn about nurturing your child's emotional health, and understand how your own childhood experiences have influenced your emotional make-up as an adult by reading or getting professional assistance.

Listed below are steps to help you booster your emotional health that were developed by Sylvia Davis of The WebMD Weight Loss Clinic. (Full article in related articles section.)

Ways to Boost Your Emotional Health

- Collect Friends

- Enjoy Solitude

- Get Fit

- Seek Pleasure

- Find a Passion

- Plan for Problems

- Seek Constructive Criticism

- Take Healthy Risks

- Manage Success Well

- Don't Go It Alone

- Write It Down

- Protect yourself from 'Energy Vampires'

Emotional health includes keeping in touch with your feelings. Sometimes girls get out of touch with their feelings and think that their feelings don't count. Some feelings are painful and really hard to deal with. Strong emotions are a signal that something in your life needs attention. The trick is figuring out what needs attention and what kind of attention it needs and providing the necessary attention to resolve the issue.

My Story: As a woman I have definitely struggled with my emotional health. We were created to feel and feel deeply, we love fast and we love hard. That has been both a benefit and a curse at some point in my life. I personally have been more concerned about the feelings of others instead of my own feelings. I have finally found a balance between the two extremes. It is very important to process your emotions completely as well as saying how you feel because, it frees you to live. The difference between emotional happiness or sadness boils down to a choice, you make the choice as to whether you will be happy or sad by your reactions to life's events. God created us as emotional beings and I am accepting of why he did it and what his expectations were for doing so. I believe that he created us to be emotional so that we would show compassion for others causing us to be the nurturers that men were not necessarily created to be. I strive daily to have optimal emotional health, some days I do other days I don't but, I will always show emotion be it good, bad or indifferent. Being true to who I am is very important to me and I hope it is to you as well. Let's look at our educational health.

Chapter 3

Educational Health-Book knowledge or No knowledge

What is Educational Health?

Educational health is based on some of the following factors:

• Critical thinking

• Problem solving

• Creativity

• Education and learning goals

• Ability to adapt to change

• Ability to access resources

• Mental status and abilities or challenges

Are you able to think about issues critically and analytically? Do you have a creative outlet in your life? Do you know what resources are available to you as a lifelong learner?

These are some essential components to your overall intellectual wellness. Once again, intellectual wellness is a vital part of your overall health and well-being.

If you want to be creative take an art class or learn a new skill. If you want to become a critical thinker, start to research both sides of an argument. Further your education, by getting a degree in an area of interest to you. Education is critical to your success in life. Everyone may not be suited for college but we are all candidates for continuous learning. You can take online classes, read or engage in intelligent conversation where you can seek knowledge from others. Get a mentor/coach who may be a field of study that interest you and glean everything you can from them to better yourself.

Sometimes people think that if you don't have a college education you are not intelligent. That could not be further from the truth. Many millionaires never went to high school let alone college. It is my belief that millionaires are born not made, there is an innate business sense that some people are just gifted with. Whether or not you have a formal education, does not make you a success or a failure. Some people are self- taught and are just as successful as the college educated. No matter what method of educating yourself you choose, just remember to be the best you can be and do everything in the spirit of excellence.

Today more and more older people are deciding to go back to school, which I think is great, Just because you get older does not mean that you stop wanting to live and learn. We all no matter the age have goals, dreams and aspirations for a better life. So just make the decision and go for it.

My Story: I personally pursued higher education, because for me I needed and wanted more out of life. I pursued my B.A. Communication and Theater with a minor in African American studies because, being a Performer was always my lifelong dream. I then decided a few years later to pursue my M.A. Counseling, Human Services and Educational Leadership with a Certification in Substance Awareness Coordination, because of my love for helping people resolve their problems by listening and then offering the necessary feedback to help them make the necessary changes in their life for the better. In June 2009 I received my B.A. in Ministry from Grace Hill Bible College. I plan on pursuing my Doctorate degree in the near future.

Just because, I decided to pursue Higher Education, does not mean I believe that everyone is destined to go to college. However, I do believe that we are to be lifelong learners whether the method is through traditional (i.e. college) or untraditional (mentorship, apprenticeship or reading). We all should strive to be become more knowledgeable for knowledge is power and it is the key to a better life. The more one learns the more marketable they become in business and in life. I am an avid reader, I read books from self-help to business, I listen to motivational CD's and I take online courses and I view educational programming. I become empowered when I learn something new and I believe it makes me a more interesting person to talk too.

Chapter 4

Relational Health-Marriage or Murder

What is Relational Health?

Relational Health is being open to creating healthy relationships with everyone in your life from your spouse to your baby-sitter.

Healthy Relationships

We all have relationships with many people in our lives and all of these relationships are different. Whether it is with friends, family, significant others, partners, acquaintances or anyone else, it is important to know how to have healthy relationships with the people in our lives. Healthy relationships increase our self-esteem, improve mental and emotional health, and help us have fuller lives.

This section focuses mostly on significant others, partners, girlfriends, boyfriends, and intimate relationships. However, most everything found here can be applied to any relationship.

Your relationships will benefit you when you learn how to communicate with your partners in a healthy way. Learn general tips on communicating, how to work out disagreements, and how to talk about sex with your partner. Check out some good feeling words to use when you're talking with people. Dating and interpersonal relationships can be confusing and take time and commitment to master.

The Question we should all ask is "Am I in a Healthy Relationship"?

Sometimes it feels impossible to find someone who's right for you and who thinks you're right for him or her! So when it happens, you're usually so psyched that you may miss some important clues into the type of person you have just encountered. It's totally normal to look at the world through rose-colored glasses in the early stages of a relationship. But for some people, those rose-colored glasses turn into blinders that keep them from seeing that a relationship isn't as healthy as it should be and maybe it's time to leave.

Have you ever asked yourself this question, what makes a Healthy Relationship? Hopefully, you and your significant other are treating each other fabulously. Not sure if that's the case? Take a step back from the dizzying sensation of being swept off your feet and think about whether your relationship has these qualities:

Mutual respect - Does he or she get how great you are and why? The key is that your spouse or significant other should be into you for who you are - for your great sense of humor, your love of reality TV, etc. Does your partner listen when you say you're not comfortable doing something and then back off right away? Respect in a relationship means that each person values whom the other is and understands - and would never challenge the other person's boundaries.

Trust - You're talking with a guy from work, and your significant other walks by. Does he completely lose his cool or keep walking because he knows you'd never cheat on him? It's OK to get a little jealous sometimes - jealousy is a natural emotion. But how a person reacts when he or she feels jealous is what matters. There's no way you can have a healthy relationship if you don't trust each other.

Honesty - This one goes hand-in-hand with trust because it's tough to trust someone who isn't being honest with you. Have you ever caught your significant other in a major lie? Like they told you that they had to work on Friday night but it turned out they were at the movies with their friends? The next time they say they have to work, you'll have a lot more trouble believing them and the trust will be on shaky ground.

Support - It's not just in bad times that your partner should support you. Some people are great when your whole world is falling apart but can't take being there when things are going right (and vice versa). In a healthy relationship, your significant other is there with a shoulder to cry on when you find out your parents are getting divorced and to celebrate with you when you accomplish one of your goals.

Fairness/equality - You need to have give-and-take relationship, too. Do you take turns choosing which new movie to see? As a couple, do you hang out with your partner's friends as often as you hang out with yours? It's not like you have to keep a running count and make sure things are exactly even, of course. But you'll know if it isn't a pretty fair balance. Things get bad really fast when a relationship turns into a power struggle, when one person is fighting to get his or her way all the time. Compromise in a relationship is a necessity. You must know that sometimes you will have to concede to win at the end, by making your spouse or significant other happy and putting their needs first.

Separate identities - In a healthy relationship, everyone needs to make compromises. But that doesn't mean you should feel like you're losing out on being yourself. When you started going out, you both had your own lives - your own families, friends, interests, hobbies, etc. - and that shouldn't change. Neither of you should have to pretend to like something you don't, give up seeing your friends, nor drop out of activities you love. And you also should feel free to keep developing new talents or interests, making new friends, and moving forward.

Good communication - You've probably heard lots of stuff about how men and women don't seem to speak the same language. We all know how many different meanings the little phrase "no, nothing's wrong" can have, depending on who's saying it! Men are from Mars and Women are truly from Venus, at least I feel that way. Men and Women speak a totally different language, but what's important is to get clarity if you're not sure what he or she means. Speak honestly and openly so that the miscommunication is avoided in the first place. Never keep your feelings bottled up because you're afraid it's not what your significant other wants to hear or because you worry about sounding silly. And if you need some time to think things through before you're ready to talk about it, take as much time as you need to and know that the right person will give you some space to do just that if you ask for it.

Just as there are healthy relationships, there are unhealthy ones as well. A relationship is unhealthy when it involves mean, disrespectful, controlling, or abusive behavior. Some people live in homes with parents who fight a lot or abuse each other - emotionally or physically. For some people who have grown up around this kind of behavior it can almost seem normal or OK. It's not! Many of us learn from watching and imitating the people close to us. So someone who has lived around violent or abusive disrespectful behavior may not have learned how to treat others with kindness and respect or how to expect the same treatment.

Qualities like kindness and respect are absolute requirements for a healthy relationship. Someone who doesn't yet have this part down may need to work on it with a trained therapist before he or she is ready for a committed relationship. Meanwhile, even though you may feel bad or feel for someone who's been mistreated, you need to take care of yourself - it's not healthy to stay in a relationship that involves abusive behavior of any kind whatsoever. If you are in such a relationship, you need to get the help and support you need to get out. You deserve to be treated like a Queen or King and nothing less. When you value yourself you make others value you as well. Relationships don't just get bad all at once; there are signs along the way, that the relationship is headed or trouble.

There are warning signs that will let you know that your relationship is an unhealthy one. Here's some scary news: In one survey, 20% of American girls reported having been hit, slapped, or forced into sexual activity by their partners. This stuff happens to guys, too - they are just less likely to report it. And 40% of all teens said they know someone at school who experienced dating violence. So if you think there's no way it could happen to you or someone you know, think again.

Ask yourself, does my spouse, boyfriend or girlfriend:

- Get angry when I don't drop everything for him or her?

- Criticize the way you look or dress?

- Do they say you'll never be able to find anyone else who would date you?

- Keep me from seeing friends or from talking to any other guys or girls?

- Want me to quit an activity, even though I love it?

- Ever raise a hand when angry, like he or she is about to hit me?

- Try to force me to go further sexually than I want to?

These aren't the only questions you can ask yourself. If you can think of any way in which your spouse, boyfriend or girlfriend is trying to control you, make you feel bad about yourself, isolate you from the rest of your world, or - this is a big one - harm you physically or sexually, then it's time to get out, fast. Let a trusted friend or family member know what's going on and make sure you're safe. It can be tempting to make excuses or misinterpret violence as an expression of love. But even if you know that the person hurting you loves you, it is not healthy. No one deserves to be hit, shoved, or forced into anything he or she doesn't want to do.

Physical, verbal or emotional abuse under no circumstances ever means LOVE, you must remember that you are too important and special to be treated any kind of way.

Ever heard about how it's hard for someone to love you when you don't love yourself? It's a big relationship roadblock when one or both people struggle with self-esteem problems. Your spouse, girlfriend or boyfriend isn't there to make you feel good about yourself if you can't do that on your own. You will need constant validation from your spouse and that's not healthy. Focus on being happy with yourself, and don't take on the responsibility of worrying about someone else's happiness. Only you can control what does or does not make you happy.

What if you feel that your spouse, girlfriend or boyfriend needs too much from you? If the relationship feels like a burden or a drag instead of a joy, it may be time to think about whether it's a healthy match for you. Someone who's not happy or secure may have trouble being a healthy relationship partner.

Relationships can be one of the best and most challenging parts of your life. They can be full of fun, romance, excitement, intense feelings, and occasional heartache, too. Whether you're single or in a relationship, remember that it's good to be choosy about whom you get close to. If you're still waiting, take your time and get to know plenty of people. Think about the qualities you value in a friendship and see how they match up with the ingredients of a healthy relationship. Work on developing those good qualities in yourself, they make you a lot more attractive to others. And if you're already part of a pair, make sure the relationship you're in brings out the best in both of you. The best thing you can do is work on you so when Mr. or Mrs. Right comes along, you will have already processed your own emotional and relationship baggage. Love and being loved is the greatest gift, it comes with a lot of responsibility, ups and down and twist and turns. Remember when you love someone love them with all that you have but don't love them to death.

My story: I have been in numerous relationships throughout my lifetime. Some of them were healthy and some were very toxic. I found it to be extremely important to find the balance between what I truly wanted and needed. Sometimes what I wanted was not what was best for me. You have to search long and hard for the characteristics your soul mate must possess and what you are flexible about. I struggled with am I good enough for him and I questioned my value a lot of the times. I would sometimes second-guess my choice in choosing my mates and sometimes I chose men who I knew were not good for me. I realized that I didn't like myself so I chose men to would exacerbate the issue by making me feel unworthy of love and happiness. I learned over the years that being in healthy relationships is very important to your total wellbeing and stability. Relationships with the others in your life are just as important as your intimate relationships. Life is about building and nurturing relationships whether they are parental, business, social or otherwise. It is important to invest time into building healthy, thriving, fulfilling relationships. I think I got it right this time, it's your turn, now enjoy the ride!

Chapter 5

Financial Health-Rich or Poor

What is Financial Health?

Financial Health is how well you handle your financial responsibilities such as budgeting, investments, credit etc.

There's never been a better time for women in particular to take control of their financial futures. Even if financial equality has not been achieved, women are more financially successful and independent than ever before. With that success comes more responsibility to organize and manage their financial health.

- There are over 10 million female-owned businesses in America, generating more than $2.5 trillion in annual revenue. (That's AWESOME!)

- Women are starting new companies at twice the rate of men, according to the National Foundation for Women Business Owners.

- Women tend to be better investors than men. According to a recent study by the National Association of Investment Clubs, women's investment clubs outperformed their male counterparts by a wide margin in 9 out of 12 years.

While more women today are taking charge of their financial future, many leave money management to men or ignore it altogether. As a result, far too many women stay on the sidelines of the money game and never take charge of their financial future.

At first glance, it may be difficult to believe that women's financial needs are all that different from men's. However, while the general principles of financial planning are universal, women face unique challenges that amount to different financial needs.

- Women live longer than men (an average of 7 years) so they need 20% more for retirement.

- On average, women earn 25% less than men.

- Since women tend to take time off to raise children or take care of parents (women take off approximately 11 years more from work than men), they save less than men do for retirement.

- After earning lower salaries for fewer years, women's social security benefits are about half of men's.

- The majority of women had certificates of deposit (CDs) in their retirement savings accounts when a more aggressive investment vehicle was more appropriate.

There are serious consequences for women who do not know how to handle their finances properly or effectively and some are as follows:

- Almost 1 in 4 women are broke within two months of a husband passing away, because they were never involved in the financial business of the family.

- Over 75% of all women are eventually widowed at an average age of 56.

- 53% of women are not covered by a pension compared to only 22% of men.

- A staggering 87% of the poverty stricken elderly are women.

The statistics are startling--but it's never too late to start taking control of your financial future.

Can't pay your bills? You're not alone. Today, millions of Americans are having difficulty paying their debts. Most of those in financial distress are middle-income families with jobs, who want to pay off what they owe.

But it is important for you to act. Doing nothing can lead to much larger problems in the future-even bigger debts, the loss of assets such as your house, and a bad credit record.

The good news is that there are solutions. The remedies provided can help improve your relationships with creditors, reduce your debts, and help you manage your money. In brief, these solutions can help give you a new, fresh start.

If bill collectors are calling you, you know you're in financial trouble. But what if you're just having difficulty stretching your paycheck to pay monthly bills? If you answer yes to any one of the following questions, you should act.

- Do you routinely spend more than you earn?

- Are you forced to make day-to-day purchases on credit?

- Are you able to make only the minimum payments on monthly credit card debts?

- If you lost your job, would you have difficulty paying next month's bills?

There are things that you can do to change your financial picture. Some tips are listed below:

Review your specific obligations that creditors claim you owe to make certain you really owe them. If you dispute a debt, first contact the creditor directly to resolve your questions. If you still have questions about the debt, contact your state or local consumer protection office or state Attorney General.

Contact your creditors to let them know you're having difficulty making your payments. Tell them why you're having trouble perhaps it's because you recently lost your job or have unexpected medical bills. Try to work out an acceptable payment schedule with your creditors. Most are willing to work with you and will appreciate your honesty and forthrightness.

The Fair Debt Collection Practices Law prohibits a debt collector from showing what you owe to anyone but your attorney, harassing or threatening you, using false statements, giving false information about you to anyone, and misrepresenting the legal status of your debts. Remember that under other federal laws to collect debts, creditors cannot seize most government assistance and can only garnish a portion of wages to collect debts.

Budget your expenses. Create a spending plan that allows you to reduce your debts. Itemize your necessary expenses (such as housing, insurance and health care) and optional expenses (such as entertainment and vacation travel). Stick to the plan.

Try to reduce your expenses. Cut out any unnecessary spending such as eating out and purchasing expensive entertainment, David Bach author of Start Late and Finish Rich calls it the Latte Factor. Consider taking public transportation rather than owning a car. Clip coupons, purchase generic products at the supermarket, and avoid impulse purchases. Above all, stop incurring new debt. Consider substituting a debit card for your credit cards. Don't spend what you don't have.

Use your savings and other assets to pay down debts. Withdrawing savings from low-interest accounts to settle high-rate loans usually makes sense. Selling off a second car not only provides cash but also reduces insurance and other maintenance expenses. Suzie Orman suggest that you only spend paper money, meaning once you break a dollar save the change and put it in a jar and see how much you can save.

Look for additional resources from governmental and private sources for which you may be eligible. Government assistance includes unemployment compensation. Aid to Families with Dependent Children (AFDC), food stamps, low-income energy assistance, Medicaid, and Social Security including disability. Other resources may be available from churches and community groups. Often these sources are listed in the Yellow Pages of your phone book.

Have you considered having your own business versus being employed?

Have you read the Rich Dad Poor Dad bestselling trilogy by Robert T. Kiyosaki? This is a must read for anyone wishing to control their financial future and even target super riches. The books in sequence are:

1.   RICH DAD POOR DAD
2.   CASHFLOW QUADRANT
3.   GUIDES TO INVESTING

Compared to a job or a self-employed profession, his presentation, rationale and arguments for building your own business are compelling. We recommend that you study his material. Here are a few quotes:

• "The rich don't work for money.... the poor and middle class works for money...the rich have money work for them."

• "A job is really a short-term solution to a long-term problem."

• "The primary reason people seek job security is because that is what they are taught to seek, at home and at school...then with debt loads, they must cling even tighter to a job, or professional security, just to pay the bills."

• "When you work hard and become successful (in a job or career), that same success brings you less and less time...even if it does bring you more money...many just burn out."

• "In moving to the business quadrant...your goal is to own a system and have people work that system for you."

• "Job security is a myth...it is also risky for self-employed people in my opinion. If they get sick, injured or die, their income is directly impacted."

- "My rich dad teaches one to focus on passive income and spend ones time acquiring the assets that provided passive or long-term residual income.... passive income from capital gains, dividends, residual income from business, rental income from real estate, and royalties."

For most of us the easiest way to produce passive income is through one of the three types below. Robert Kiyosaki outlines three types of businesses:

1. A startup corporation - where you develop your own system
2. Franchises - where you buy an existing system
3. Network Marketing - where you buy into and become part of the existing system (for example Youngevity, Soul Purpose, nSpire Network, Total Life Changes, just to name a few.

The first two are the most risky, require the most capital and skills and are therefore beyond the average person. There are huge leverage advantages for the individual within the structure of a good network marketing company. For more information on home based businesses, network marketing and business opportunities, you can contact me directly via my website at www.mrsopportunity.info or you may e-mail me at diamondenterprisesinc@yahoo.com. I personally LOVE network marketing and I have been involved in the industry for a number of years now and I would not change a thing.

You may be asking, what is the purpose of my own business? The development of your own business represents the development of an asset (an asset is defined by Robert Kiyosaki as a vehicle that produces income). A business asset produces passive income i.e. it does not require your daily effort to produce the income. Passive income increases from the growth of your business and from increased tax sheltering of income available to business enterprises. Sheltered surplus income should be reinvested within the business structure to create other forms of investment with passive income also. In simple terms, this is the method used by the mega-rich to accumulate their assets. You have to decide what you want financially and get a financial advisor to help you with your financial goals and create a plan of action.

My Story: I constantly struggle in this area. I am not a millionaire yet but I am working on it by building both traditional and network marketing businesses. It seems that there is never enough money to meet my needs or philanthropic/humanitarian desires. I realized after being burdened with credit card debt as a college student, that spending cash was far better than spending plastic. The credit card industry draws you in and then squashes you by hitting you with every imaginable and unimaginable credit card charge. By the time you realize it, you are knee deep in debt. I have been there, done that and I don't wish the bill collector harassment on anyone. I have learned over the years that I must only spend what I can afford to. It is better to wait to get something you want when you can afford it, than to be in debt for the rest of your life. Your credit score is crucial to your financial health. The better your score the better your financial choices. Now let's look at social health.

Chapter 6

Social Health-Friend or Friendless

What is Social Health?

Social well-being is a very important part in creating and maintaining a balanced and healthy lifestyle. Just think back to a difficult time in your life.... did it make it better knowing that you had the support, consideration and encouragement from a strong social network?

Some components of social wellness include:

- The caring and healthy relationships you have in your life.

- Your social networks, such as what clubs and/or organizations you belong to.

- Your level of safety.

- Your housing situation.

- Your level of interdependence, and if you are willing to accept and give help to other people.

- Positive interactions with your community (i.e. volunteer work).

- Your acceptance of diversity. This means accepting people regardless of their ethnicity, gender, sexual orientation, ability or religion. Students may become so overwhelmed with school that you neglect this part of your well-being. Just remember that your connection to your friends, family and community is important in maintaining balance in your day-to-day life.

The concept of social health is less intuitively familiar than that of physical or mental health, and yet, along with physical and mental health, it forms one of the three pillars of most definitions of health. This is partly because social health can refer both to a characteristic of a society, and of individuals. "A society is healthy when there is equal opportunity for all and access by all to the goods and services essential to fully function as a citizen". Indicators of the health of a society might include the existence of the rule of law, equality in the distribution of wealth, public accessibility of the decision making process, and the level of social capital.

The social health of individuals refers to "that dimension of an individual's well-being that concerns how he gets along with other people, how other people react to him and how he interacts with social institutions and societal mores".

This definition is broad—it incorporates elements of personality and social skills, reflects social norms, and bears a close relationship to concepts such as "well-being," "adjustment," and "social functioning."

Formal consideration of social health was stimulated in 1947 by its inclusion in the World Health Organization's definition of health, and by the resulting emphasis on treating patients as social beings who live in a complex social context. Social health has also become relevant with the increasing evidence that those who are well integrated into their communities tend to live longer and recover faster from disease. Conversely, social isolation has been shown to be a risk factor for illness. Hence, social health may be defined in terms of social adjustment and social support—or the ability to perform normal roles in society.

Mutual social support is also commonly viewed as an aspect of social health. Support attenuates the effects of stress and reduces the incidence of disease. Social support also contributes to positive adjustment in children and adults, and encourages personal growth. The concept of support underlines the theme of social health as an attribute of a society: a sense of community—or the currently fashionable concept of social capital, which refers to the extent to which there is a feeling of mutual trust and reciprocity in a community—is an important indicator of social health.

It is important to be socially accepted in the community in which you live, work and play. Being able to adapt in various social situations could very well mean the difference between being included or excluded from the group. Sometimes people feel like outcast in social situations because, they were not taught proper social skills when they were growing up. Parents need to teach their children how to behave in social situations, so that when they reach adulthood, they are well adjusted to these social environments.

My Story: I have found that over the years, my social health has increased. My social health in college was excellent but it decreased after graduate school. I became somewhat introverted and preferred to be a homebody instead of a social butterfly. Within the past couple of years I have become more social by necessity as well as by desire. I have enjoyed the interaction with other people for the most part. I find that I like being in the company of people who have a similar mindset or goals as I do. I am drawn to driven, goal oriented, self-motivated, and energetic people more than to people who have no direction, dreams or desires.

No matter what anyone may say, we all need people in our lives and just want to be loved and accepted by others. In this age of technology, we must not forget the importance of verbal communication.

The next section deals with issues concerning the body, which include physical and environmental health. Physical health is what most people think about when someone asks them how they are doing? Or when we think about our health, we automatically think physical. Then we will view what environmental health is all about and how it relates to the body.

Chapter 7

Physical Health – Life or Death

What is Physical Health?

"Physical health is the overall condition of a living organism at a given time, the soundness of the body, freedom from disease or abnormality, and the condition of optimal well-being. People want to function as designed, but environmental forces can attack the body or the person may have genetic malfunctions. The main concern in health is preventing injury and healing damage caused by injuries and biological attacks." Ron Kurtus (revised 22 September 2002 www. school-for-champions.com}

Questions you may have about what health is include:

• How does health relate to the function of the body?

• What about getting sick or injured?

• How is healing related to health?

Each one of us was born with a body that is a highly complex mechanism. It is amazing that it operates as well as it does. Good health is really defined as being able to function according to the way the body has been designed to function.

Unfortunately, no one is perfect and many people have defects in their bodies. Some people have defects that can be life-threatening. Fortunately, the body can compensate for defects and a person may easily live a long life with a body that is only partially functioning. An example is how a blind person or crippled person can compensate for the handicap and simply turn it into a challenge and win.

Not only should all the body parts work well and work together, they also need proper nutrition for energy and to continue to operate effectively. In general, humans and animals seem to be able to tell what foods their bodies need to function properly and to be healthy. Unfortunately, there are foods that can be harmful, but yet fool the brain in saying they are good for you. At the extreme, there are addictive drugs. But there are also salty, fatty, and sugary food that both humans and animals' love, but that can be harmful to the health and nutritional needs of the being. ." Ron Kurtus (revised 22 September 2002 www.school-for-champions.com}

Exercise is an important component in relation to our physical health. If you have a Porsche sports car, it does no good to be driving it to and from the laundry mat or running your daily errands. The car was made for the high speeds of the open roads. Likewise with your body, it was made to be used and therefore should be on a regular basis.

The human body was made to be physically active not sedentary like a couch potato. The heart needs to pump fast once in a while to keep its muscle tone. Your lungs need exercise to function the way they were made to function. Exercise and using the body is important to maintaining your health.

Sickness affects our physical beings by way of germs, bacteria, molds, and viruses, which may attack parts of our bodies, trying to infiltrate and use the body as a home or source of food. Not only can they destroy our cells, but also they often may release poisons that can harm our whole being. ." Ron Kurtus (revised 22 September 2002 www.schoolfor-champions.com}

Cleanliness is one defense against disease. Also, the body creates internal defenses against specific bacteria and viruses. In fact, because the body builds up these defenses, there is a question whether being too clean is actually good for you, because you may then not develop the natural defenses needed to maintain your health. ." Ron Kurtus (revised 22 September 2002 www.school-for-champions.com}

Injury to parts of our body can come from attacks by animals or other people, or they can occur through an accident. Caution is the best defense against injury. Carelessness or ignorance often results in injury. ." Ron Kurtus (revised 22 September 2002 www.school-for-champions.com}

A major part of health concerns healing. After you have become sick or injured, your body will fight the disease and then attempt to heal the wounds. Although there are some drugs that can relieve pain, the major part of healing is natural. Protecting against further attacks or injury and being in good health helps the healing process. Being in good physical condition is critical to your overall health and wellness; this is where physical activity comes into play.

Physical activity' is a term that describes any movement involving large muscles. Running, walking, cycling, skipping, swimming, dancing and playing all types of sports are all kinds of physical activity. Taking part in a sport, recreation or other physical activities need not be taken seriously. Casual but regular participation will achieve benefits. Walking id one of the very best forms of physical activity and anyone can do it For FREE!

You may ask yourself, WHY SHOULD I BE PHYSICALLY ACTIVE? Physical activity has a range of important health and social benefits. Research has found that middle-aged men who began exercising at a moderate intensity had an improved life expectancy and a reduced risk of coronary heart disease, even when other risk factors (smoking, high blood pressure and being overweight) are present. It is important to maintain a significant level of activity throughout life to stay healthy. Even if you were fit when you were younger you don't retain the low risk profile that you once had. For those who have been inactive in their youth, it is never too late to become physically active and gain a significant health benefit.

NATIONAL PHYSICAL ACTIVITY GUIDELINES

These guidelines refer to the minimum levels of physical activity that is required for good health. They are not intended for high levels of fitness or sports training. Try to carry out the guidelines and for the best results combine an active lifestyle with healthy eating.

1. THINK OF MOVEMENT AS AN OPPORTUNITY NOT AN INCONVENIENCE

Modern technology has reduced much of our need for movement. Cars now reduce our need for walking, machines do the heavy work for us, and technology such as TVs, computers, and videos keep us inactive for long periods of time. This decrease in activity has been associated with an increase in obesity and other health problems. We have embraced the benefits of this technology and now consider 'unnecessary' movement an inconvenience. It is necessary to change these attitudes towards movement. It is possible to enjoy the benefits of modern technology without negative health consequences.

2. BE ACTIVE EVERYDAY IN AS MANY WAYS AS YOU CAN

Research has found that even the most inactive people can gain health benefits if they become even slightly more active. Small increases in daily activity come from small changes carried out throughout the day. For example, making a habit of walking or cycling to the store, doing some gardening, parking your car a little further away and/or doing things by hand instead of using labor saving devices.

3. PUT TOGETHER AT LEAST 30 MINUTES OF MODERATE-INTENSITY PHYSICAL ACTIVITY ON MOST, PREFERABLY ALL, DAYS

Improvements in health indicators- such as blood pressure, blood cholesterol and body weight- can result from doing 30 minutes of activity each day.

Moderate-intensity activity will cause a slight, but noticeable increase in breathing and heart rate. An example of a moderate intensity activity is a brisk walk at a pace where you can comfortably talk but not sing. Other examples include mowing the lawn, medium paced swimming or cycling.

4. IF YOU CAN, ENJOY SOME REGULAR, VIGOROUS ACTIVITY FOR EXTRA HEALTH AND FITNESS

This guideline doesn't replace earlier recommendations it adds an extra level for those who are able to, and who wish to achieve greater health and fitness benefits. Children and teenagers should follow this guideline routinely. Vigorous' implies activity, which makes you 'huff and puff', and where talking in full sentences between breaths are difficult. Vigorous activity includes active sports i.e. jogging, football, squash, netball or aerobics.

Physical activity is a MUST if you want to maintain optimal health and wellness.

HEALTH BENEFITS

Participation in regular physical activity improves health in a number of ways.

Here are just a few:

- Extends life and reduces the risk of premature death.

- Improves blood cholesterol.

- Relieves moderate depression and stress.

- Favorably affects blood pressure.

- Helps maintain healthy body weight.

- Reduces the risk of developing diabetes.

BARRIERS

Many people feel that there are barriers that prevent them from starting a physical activity program. These can include:

Time – You can improve your level of physical activity even if time is limited. Look for easy ways to be more active throughout the day.

Age – Regular physical activity is associated with a 40% decreased risk of losing mobility for older people. (Active Australia 2000). This means a better quality of life, protection against accidental falls as well as stronger bones and muscles. Moderate activities include walking, swimming, gardening, playing golf and even energetic housework!

Travel – Many hotels and motels have fitness centers that are available for guests to use. Some of the larger hotels also provide walking and jogging maps, which are a great way of getting out and doing some sightseeing at the same time as getting some exercise.

The weather – If it's cold outside dress appropriately and take a brisk walk. Utilize the local heated swimming pool or look for opportunities to play indoor team sports. If the weather is hot, again try the swimming pool or walk or ride early in the mornings or evenings when it's cooler.

A major part of your life is your physical health. Good physical health can contribute to leading a satisfying and successful life. There are factors involved in having satisfying physical health. Three principles to follow that will improve your chances for a healthy life are to be physically active, be nutritionally prudent, and minimize medical involvement

Questions you may have include:

*   What is the value of activity?

*   Why worry about what I eat?

*   Why minimize medial involvement??

The expression goes "use it or lose it." If you do not use your muscles, lungs and heart as much as they were intended to be used, they will atrophy (waste away).

Exercise can provide many benefits such as keeping your system working properly, keeping your weight at a healthy level, giving you more energy and endurance, allowing you to bounce back quicker from injury or disease, and generally maintaining your health.

Your activity must be regular. You cannot expect to make up for a weeks of inactivity with a spurt of exercise on one Saturday.

Overkill of anything is not healthy. You should be practical in what you eat. Studies show that animals and people who eat less live longer. But of course, that does not mean eating so little that you become anorexic. It is my belief that one should eat between 3 to 6 meals per day to ensure that the body is getting the nutrients it desires.

Also try to eat more healthy foods, like fruits, vegetables and whole grains just name a few. Eating junk foods or those high in animal fat is not a nutritional sound diet. Remember what Benjamin Franklin wrote in his Poor Richard's Almanac: "An apple a day keeps the doctor away." That is good advice that can be extended to other nutritional foods. If you eat a well-balanced diet, you will be well on your way to a healthy body. Remember you are what you eat and everything you put in your mouth will show up one way or the other.

Also be careful when you see a doctor. Remember that medicine is a business and sometimes doctors prescribe what is convenient to them instead of the patient and that they are trying to figure out what will help you, they really are practicing and learning as they go along. You need to be an active participant in your health and wellness. Don't be afraid to ask your doctor questions about your conditions, if you have any. Avoid drugs and operations unless absolutely necessary. Often they can do more harm than good. In general, use caution when being medically treated and get a second opinion if necessary. You and your doctors are partners in your healthcare, but you do have the final say.

Most of us know the impact that stress, depression, or euphoria can have on our bodies. Can profound physical problems really be related to the way we feel and think? Most of us have experienced the physical effects that depression, mental strain or stress can have on our bodies, or the euphoria of a really good day that makes every ache or pain feel better. We know that sleep can have an impact on our minds and emotions as well as our physical energy levels. In fact, our emotions are fundamentally connected with all aspects of health.

The link between mental, emotional and physical health has been gaining credibility ever since Louise Hay brought the concept into the public eye over two decades ago. Her books You Can Heal Your Body and You Can Heal Your Life are the modern foundation for the kind of healing that looks at our lives from a holistic or "whole being" perspective. Our health, illness, and even the shapes of our bodies have been linked to mental and emotional patterns that create implications in our physical reality over time.

"Neither our bodies, minds, heart, nor spirit exist in a vacuum: each is fundamentally dependent on the others in order for us to be healthy and whole. This concept is hardly new. In traditional human societies, emotional well-being would have been the purvey of the shaman, wise woman, medicine man, or healer - the same person who knew how to heal and improve physical health." (Victoria Anisman-Reiner, June 10, 2006).

In today's world, many natural medicine practitioners are able to help clients release emotional strain, phobias, and ingrained habits, even as they treat physical allergies and other symptoms. Even ordinary physical symptoms may end up being traced to painful memories or experiences that have become locked in the body's energy field and need to be released or reframed. Healers using techniques like cranial sacral, deep body massage, energy medicine or energy psychology are able to use physical tools to clear emotional blocks and trauma quickly, enabling people to walk away after just one or two sessions with less pain, fear - and decreased physical symptoms." (Victoria Anisman-Reiner, June 10, 2006).

What kind of physical problems have been linked to emotional well-being? The most common ones, stomachache and headache, can be caused by virtually any kind of strain. Back pain has been attributed to a feeling of not being emotionally supported, or to feeling that you've lost your path or aren't fulfilling your purpose. Knee problems can be due to fear of "stepping forward" in your life. Asthma, especially in childhood, has been linked to a feeling of smothering or too much control. Cancer is related to self-hatred, and fibromyalgia and other degenerative diseases to a deep feeling of unworthiness and abnegation of self. Thyroid has to do with the voice, expressing yourself and feeling that you are heard.

Our bodies manifest illness to show our thoughts and feelings. They can truly be our greatest teachers about what is going on inside our hearts and minds... and how to heal us.

"Physical activity improves health and well-being. It reduces stress, strengthens the heart and lungs, increases energy levels, helps you maintain and achieve a healthy body weight and it improves your outlook on life."(Lerche Davis. Jeanie Aug. 2, 2001}

Research shows that physical inactivity can cause premature death, chronic disease and disability.

For children, regular physical activity is essential for healthy growth and development. For adults, it allows daily tasks to be accomplished with greater ease and comfort and with less fatigue. For seniors, weight-bearing physical activity reduces the rate of bone loss associated with osteoporosis and regular physical activity maintains strength and flexibility, balance and coordination and can help reduce the risk of falls. Regular physical activity prolongs independent living. Being physically active not only strengthens your body -- it also makes you feel good about yourself.

There is so much that can be done to get physical activity in your life. Bodily movement is something that everyone can do on a regular basis. It is not necessary to run a marathon or spend time at a gym unless that is your preference. All you need to do is find uncomplicated ways to be physically active every day.

What you could do is:

- Take a walk during your lunch period.

- Take the stairs instead of the elevator.

- Get from in front of the television or computer.

- Play with your children.

- Get a workout video.

- Get buddy to workout with.

- Walk or ride a bike instead of driving.

- Jump rope.

- Park your car farther and walk more.

- Participate in gardening.

- Do housework.

- Dance, dance, dance.

- Just move daily.

Stress and health are closely linked. It is well known that stress, either chronic or acute, can encourage risky body mind disorders. Disorders such as dizzy spells, anxiety, tension, sleeplessness, nervousness and muscle cramps can all result in chronic health problems. In the long run they may also affect our bodies other systems.

There are variable thoughts on whether stress actually has any impact on our cardiovascular system or not. However, there is research that shows that in certain individuals stress does contribute to high blood pressure, high cholesterol, and other cardiac risk factors such as addictions and obesity. Stress induced or not, suffering from cardiac conditions is in itself quite stressful for most individuals and their families.

Still physical causes of stress such as vigorous physical activity and exercises can place demands on the heart muscle of the weak or of people already suffering from coronary blockage. It is evident that people who live in chronically stressed-out conditions are more likely to take up smoking, alcohol and substance abuse (drugs, prescribed or illegal), fall into eating disorders (unhealthy food habits) and inertia. Medical practitioners say all of these stress-related behaviors have a direct effect on the development of coronary artery diseases. It is extremely important to consultant your doctor, before beginning any exercise program especially if you are currently under a doctor's care.

My Story: My journey to physical wellness has definitely had its ups, downs and turnarounds to say the least. It's been challenging, frustrating and truly disappointing at times. My weight has fluctuated since I can remember. I suffered from high blood pressure until I decided to make a change and do something about it. I knew that I was not being a physically active as I needed and I enlisted some help. I joined gyms, paid for them and didn't go; I bought videos and DVDs, paid for them and didn't use them. It was not until I got sick and tired of wasting my hard earned money that I knew I had to make a serious commitment to change my life by losing weight and becoming physically fit.

I have done better over the years; it is a lifelong process, but I feel better, look better and act better as a result of better, improved overall physical health. I am still struggling as I am writing this book, I have good days and I have bad days but most importantly I have healthy days. I have changed my eating habits for the better, I eat everything in moderation, and I don't deprive myself of the foods I like. I have found new, healthy and delicious ways to prepare my food. I am determined to reach my goal by my next birthday. I know that the older you get the harder it get to lose the weight. I am determined to be in the best physical condition I possibly can be and to live the live the life I was designed, created and destined to. I have a vision of what the perfect physical me looks like and I won't stop until I reach my goal. I know that I will have setbacks but I will not use them as crutches or excuses not to continue what I started. I found this great new program called The Diet free Life System and I absolutely love it. It has helped me begin a program that I can live with for the rest of my life because simply, I love food and I will be a food lover for life. Visit http://www.dietfreelife.com for more information. I have not reached my goal yet, but I will not stop trying until I accomplish my goal and reach my goal weight. I continue to read books and view workout programs to find solutions to my problem. I am more than a conqueror and I will be a winner, physically and in every area of my life. If you are ready to begin your physical journey we can do this together. I am a big advocate of pampering to de-stress to lessen the attack on the physical body. I have been involved in Aromatherapy for some time now and it has changed my life, it not only has helped my body but it has helped my mind as well.

Chapter 8

Environmental Health – Safe or Hazardous

What is Environmental Health?

Environmental health simply put is the wellness of our surroundings from where we live, work and play. There are many infractions, which create bad environmental health.

Ingesting the wrong material can poison a person. Sometimes poisons are subtle parts of the environment, such as smog or drugs. Being aware of potential poisons is an important defense. Sometimes environmental poisoning is unavoidable, since you may not even realize it is happening to you. In many communities, people spread poisons on their lawns to kill insects and then let their children play on the lawn, often resulting in problems years down the road. It is a fact that our bodies are constantly under attack from our environment.

Sometimes it is under attack even from us. It is our responsibility to save the planet from destruction, by doing whatever we can individually as well as collectively to ensure a long happy life.

The toxins in our environment greatly attribute to the seriousness of the illnesses that we have contracted with no cure. Our children are subjected to toxins at school because of the chemicals used in the industrial cleaning products. Pollution, dust, and smog etc., are all contributors to our unsafe environment. Improper garbage disposal, contaminated water systems all add to a disease-ridden culture. We all must be active participants in the fight for environmental equality and safety.

As parents, it is our responsibility to protect our children from all things. Environmental health usually slips behind the radar. The chemicals we use in our homes can cause the illnesses that our children suffer from. We must educate ourselves, so that we can educate our children, so that we can create a healthier, better world around us. Global Warming is a very serious thing and we all must be active participants in our own Environmental Health. There are many products on the market today, which can definitely assist us in making the necessary changes because everyone can do something. We must all make the sacrifice to have safe the planet.

My story: I have just learned over the last couple years about the toxins that I encountered in my daily living and I have since made healthier, safer choices about the household & personal products I use. I have personally removed a great number of the unsafe toxic products from my home & personal care regimen. I have switched to better environmentally safe products for the home like Atomy, Youngevity and some online brands just to name a few. And I have changed to healthier nature based personal care products from Soul Purpose, Warm Spirit etc. Because of my need to use better, safer products I decided to create my own line of products called Just Make Scents. By switching products, I believe I am doing my part to help the environment last a little longer for my children's, children and generations to come. Everyone can do his or her part in saving our environment, so why don't you join me by making a change for the better TODAY! Start with one thing at a time and keep making small changes and trust me you will be glad you did. It will not only help you and your family but it will be a help to our world.

Chapter 9

Spiritual Health – Victor or Victim

What is Spiritual Health?

Spiritual health is the way you find meaning, hope, comfort and inner peace in your life. Many people find spirituality through religion. Some find it through music, art or a connection with nature. Others find it in their values and principles.

Spiritual health is unique to each individual. Your "Spirit" usually refers to the deepest part of you, the part that lets you make meaning of your world. Your spirit provides you with the revealing sense of who you are, why you are here and what your purpose for living is. It is that innermost part of you that allows you to gain strength and hope.

Spiritual wellness may not be something that you think much of, yet its impact on your life is unavoidable. The basis of spirituality is discovering a sense of meaningfulness in your life and coming to know that you have a purpose to fulfill.

What does it mean to be spiritual? Here are a few ideas... It means you're experiencing unity, making things whole, or feeling "at one with." It's about building bridges. It's about love. To live spiritually means that you're making positive connections, connections within yourself, with other people, with God, or with the world around you (self-renewal.com, 2006).

For some, spirituality may be equated with traditional religions such as Christianity, Hinduism or Buddhism. For others, it may mean growing in your personal relationships with others, or through being at peace with nature.

Assessing Your Spiritual Health

Where are you at in your spiritual life? Take a moment to reflect…do you feel a sense of worth, hope, purpose, commitment or peace? Do you have a positive outlook on life? Or do you experience feelings of emptiness, anxiety, hopelessness, apathy or conflict? These may be signs of spiritual poverty in your life and may be the reason for unhappiness or dissatisfaction.

Many wellness behaviors can benefit your spiritual health. Such behaviors include feeling connected with others, feeling part of a community, volunteering, having an optimistic attitude, contributing to society and self -love/care.

Here are some ways to help improve your spiritual health:

•   Be quiet. Take time for yourself every day, even if it's just before you go to sleep, or when you're driving home.

•   Be open. Spiritual experiences can happen anywhere at any time.

•   Practice being non-judgmental and having an open mind

- Be receptive to pain or times of sorrow. It is often in these times when we discover how spirituality can help us cope.

- Practice forgiveness

- Pray, meditate or worship

- Live joyfully

- Allow yourself to believe in things, that aren't easily explainable.

No one really knows for sure how spirituality is related to health. However, it seems the body, mind and spirit are connected. The health of any one of these elements seems to affect the health of the others. Some research shows that things such as positive beliefs, comfort and strength gained from religion, meditation and prayer can contribute to healing and a sense of well-being. Improving your spiritual health may not cure an illness, but it may help you feel better, prevent some health problems and help you cope with illness or death.

If you want to improve your spiritual health, you may want to try the following ideas. Remember, though, that everyone is different, so what works for others may not work for you. Do what is comfortable for you.

- Identify the things in your life that give you a sense of inner peace, comfort, strength, love and connection.

- Set aside time every day to do the things that help you spiritually. These may include doing community service or volunteer work, praying, meditating, singing devotional songs, reading inspirational books, taking nature walks, having quiet time for thinking, d playing a sport or attending religious services.

If you are being treated for an illness, it's important for your doctor to know how your spirituality might be affecting your feelings and thoughts about your medical situation. If you think your spiritual beliefs are affecting your health care decisions or your ability to follow your doctor's recommendations, tell your doctor.

If you have spiritual beliefs, worries or concerns that are causing you stress, talk with your doctor. Your doctor would like to help. If your doctor can't help you with these issues, he or she may be able to suggest someone who can.

What is more important: Physical Health, or Spiritual Health?

For an agnostic, this is obviously a moot point, however a believer is very likely concerned about both. But, how does God feel about people's Physical and Spiritual Health?

When the Preacher asked the congregation how many wanted to go to Heaven, everyone's hand went up. When he asked how many wanted to go right now, most of the hands stayed down.

When faced with the reality of suddenly leaving the world behind, even to some believers, all that unfinished, earthly business seems to be more important than meeting one's maker. However, for believers and non-believers alike - the time will come when everyone's spirit will return to Him who gave it and await judgment by Jesus Christ, the Son of God (John 5: 22; Ro 14:10).

At that time, the rich and poor, the healthy and sick, the beautiful and the homely, the wise and ignorant - will all meet on common ground, and everyone's actions, comments, and faithfulness either in the law, or without the law, will be judged and weighed against one's motives, and between the time spent for God and for oneself (De 18:19, John 12:48, Mat 7:2, 22-23, Mat 12:36-37, 1Co 3:11-15, Ro 2:12-16, Just like some people who are obsessed with accumulating riches, or spending every free minute in the gym to sculpture that perfect body, or go through the most stringent dietary rituals for optimal health, God is so obsessed for an individual to be redeemed that he only allows for two choices - saved and unsaved. Nothing in between which forces every individual not to be complacent about his or her own destiny.

How concerned is God about good health and nutrition?

In some early books of the Old Testament, God instructed his people on how to cultivate the land, and cautioned them about unclean foods, including the adverse consequences of touching dead, diseased, or infectious humans and animals, or using contaminated utensils.

He spoke unfavorably against gluttony and drunkenness. While it is unknown whether there had ever been a time when vegetarianism was prevalent, eating meat throughout the Old and New Testament was neither a sin, nor spoken against, with Jesus Himself not only eating fish, but also meat, the Passover lamb being one example. The apostle Paul only admonished to abstain from meat (and wine) if it were to cause another believer to stumble or be offended, or made weak (Romans 14:21).

There have been occasions in the Scriptures where God struck some individuals with a particular disease for their deeds (Numbers 12:1-10, 2 Kings 5:27, 2Chronicles 21:12-15, 2Chronicles 26:18-20). Some believers were said to have been weak and sickly because of unworthily taking part in sacraments (1Co 11:27-30). Others were sick because of sin (Micah 6:13), wine (Hosea 7:5), love / lust (2Samuel 13:1-2), prophetic visions (Daniel 8:27), accidents (2Samuel 4:4), or afflictions attributed to Satan (Job 2:7, Luke 13:1116).

Not all who were - or are sick now, are suffering as a result of divine punishment for their sins: When asked why a particular man was blind from birth - whether it was as a result of him, or his parents sinning - Jesus answered, Neither hath this man sinned, nor his parents: but that the works of God should be made manifest in him.˜ (John 9:3, also John 11:4) - which illustrates that God places greater emphasis on the eternal benefits of spiritual health, rather than the transient benefits of physical health.

How important is prayer?

Prayer is a form of spiritual communication with the Holy Trinity for Praise, Worship, Thanksgiving, and Repentance, and it provides a means of communicating our desire for God to bless and fulfill the needs of others and to bring any concerns we have before the Lord for spiritual guidance.

Daily prayer establishes a relationship with God through the Lord Jesus Christ, which is a requisite for forgiveness of sins and salvation (John 14:6, Col 1:14, Romans 10:9), and it provides emotional comfort and spiritual strength to withstand life's trials and tribulations, while the Holy Ghost empowers believers to bear fruit of the spirit. Unfortunately, a lot of people think of prayer only as a petition to help them achieve a particular goal, or they use prayer only during a crisis. Before Jesus taught his disciples how to pray, he assured them: ...for your Father knoweth what things ye have need of, before ye ask him.~ (Matthew 6:8), and " But seek ye first the kingdom of God, and his righteousness; and all these things shall be added unto you (Matthew 6:33)."

Do people get healed through prayer?

There are Biblical accounts where prayers for healing were answered (2 Kings 20, 1-7, Acts 28:8), and the apostle James wrote to 'let the elders of the church pray over the sick, and anoint them with oil in the name of the Lord' (Jas 5:14-15), however I am not aware of any Scriptural passages which suggest that prayer alone - in the absence of someone anointed with the gift of healing (1Co 12:9) - would heal the sick. In fact, the apostle Paul, who had received the gift of healing, was denied to overcome his own infirmities (2 Corinthians 12:7-10), and those of Timothy (1Timothy 5:23).

Many people confuse spiritual healing with physical health or healing. Jesus said ...Take no thought for your life, what ye shall eat, or what ye shall drink; ~ (Matthew 6:25), which - if applied to physical health - would challenge every facet of medical research that has shown a link between good nutrition and better health. The spiritual aspect of the physical healings Jesus performed is further demonstrated when He rebuked some of the scribes and said: Whether is it easier to say to the sick of the palsy, Thy sins be forgiven thee; or to say, Arise, and take up thy bed, and walk (Mark2: 9).

Spiritual health comes with our sincere devotion to the Creator with prayers, reading of the Bible or other instruction manual for living and being in the company of the good people. We all should be concerned about our spiritual health and well-being. May God keep us all in good physical, mental and spiritual health.

Spiritual people, particularly those who attend religious services, may live longer, healthier lives than others, according to two recent studies.

One study, from the University of Texas at Austin, stresses the role of regular religious attendance — not just spirituality — in longevity and general health. This study found that people who attend religious services one or more times a week live to an average age of 83 — an average of eight years longer than those who never attend church.

Researchers on this study suggest that the healthful effects of religious attendance may be related to the lifestyle choices that many churchgoers are likely to make, including the social ties that are often developed among congregation members.

This study, from the Population Research Center at the university, was published in the May 1999 issue of the journal Demography. A second study, from the Georgia Baptist Family Practice Residency Program, agreed that people who described themselves as highly or moderately spiritual were generally healthier than those who reported low levels of spirituality. This research was published in the February 1998 issue of the journal Family Medicine.

Dr. Chandrakant Shah, professor of public health sciences at the University of Toronto, has been reviewing statistical data from Canada's National Population Health Survey. He feels certain that spirituality provides those who practice it health benefits of reduced stress, improved social connectedness, and healthier lifestyles -- all of which are well-known factors in lowering mortality. Dr. Shah defines spirituality as the beliefs and values one holds concerning one's place in the universe and which reflect one's connections with a higher power and social and physical environments. Dr. Shah recommends a balanced approach to material achievement, respect for the environment, volunteer work and caring for family and friends as individual measures to help with spirituality. No matter what your spiritual belief may be, it is necessary to have one.

My story: I have believed in God all of my life and was raised in the church. I know that without him I would be nothing and I would surely fail. We were created in his image and we must duplicate his life as we journey through life. For me it was crucial to have a Heavenly Father in my life, which I could turn too, when human flesh let me down. God is my rock and my refuge, my very present help in the times of trouble. We were created to serve others and as we give to others we will surely gain beyond measure. For me spiritual wellness is the catalyst to all these other forms of wellness. I struggle daily in this area because, it is hard to live in a word of unbelievers all around and not have some doubts. The one thing I know for sure is that we all should believe in a Divine Power higher than our own.

I have questioned on occasion whether God is listening to me as I pray and I began to realize, of course he is because I have made it to see another day. I honor God for keeping me daily during the perilous times we are living in. I try to show gratitude for everything that he has given to and done for me. God is the center of my joy and without him I would surely die. As a way to get closer to God and fulfill my purpose, I became a licensed Evangelist/Missionary in July 2009 and I received my B.A. in Ministry in June 2009 and my M.A. in Christian Education.

God is my father, my best friend, my counselor, and my provider; simply put God is my EVERYTHING! I will serve him for the rest of my life.

Chapter 10

Conclusion – It's all up to you!

Health is when your body functions as it is supposed to. Wellness is having BALANCE in your life. You need nutrition and exercise to maintain your health. Your body defends itself against illness and disease, but you must use caution to avoid injury and poisonous substances. If you are healthy, you will heal quicker.

Each day you make many decisions that affect your happiness, wholeness & wellness. For example, you may decide to use a seat belt, to drink milk instead of soda, or go to sports practice. While each of these decisions may seem small, taken together, day after day and year after year, they have a big effect on your life. They influence your daily energy level and self-confidence, as well as your future health & wellness.

It is not always easy to take the action necessary to create change. However, without taking some action, you cannot make changes in your life that may be necessary to help you feel better. Every time you take a positive step in creating change in your life, give yourself a pat on the back or reward yourself by doing something nice for yourself like taking a warm bath by candlelight, going for a walk, or spending some time with a friend. You also may want to keep a written record of the changes you are creating in your life in a notebook or journal.

Making changes takes time and may be difficult. You may have to overcome many obstacles. Take small steps. Don't give up.

Be persistent. Keep working toward whatever it is that will help you to feel better and enjoy your life more. Making changes is being able to see beyond you to seeing what the solution might be.

Creating change is something you need to do for yourself. No one else can do it for you. Others can help you and support you as you create change but it is up to you to do what needs to be done. You will be the one that benefits from successful change.

When thinking about health and fitness, focus on the three Cs: centered, committed, and consistent.

1. You need to get CENTERED.

Gather yourself, your thoughts, and think about what you want out of life.

2. You have to make a true COMMITMENT.

You can accomplish anything that you set your mind to. Take a stand for yourself and commit to making those changes you want to see in yourself.

3. Understand it takes CONSISTENCY, and make it happen.

You'll hit bumps along the road. When this happens, get right back to it. Consistency doesn't mean perfection. It means staying true to the cause, and never giving up.

If you need help accomplishing any of your wellness goals, I suggest you do what I did. I found a coach to help me focus my life, support me in my own personal journey and hold me accountable. A coach helps me be accountable for the goals I set, the commitments I make and most importantly they help me direct my life and reclaim my power which allows me to live a life of authenticity and greatness. And yes I am a coach and coaches need coaches too. Visit http://bit.ly/bewelltoday if you decide that you want to consider working with me.

Today is the beginning of the best days of your life, embrace it, love it and live it fully. Take control of your choices and choose to LIVE YOUR BEST LIFE, FROM THE INSIDE OUT!

Suggestions for Improving Your Life

Suggestions for better mental health:

    Don't give away your power

    Learn to relax, relate and release

    Meditate

Suggestions for better emotional health:

    Learn how to manage your emotions

    Choose your battles

    Learn how to cope with life's changes

    Share your feelings

Suggestions for better educational health:

    Enroll in school

    Take a training course in any area of interest to you

    Read, read and read some more

    Engage in meaningful conversations

    Become a self –learner

Suggestions for better social health:

Join civic or community groups

Be approachable

Go to networking events

Practice developing social skills

Interact with people from other cultures

Suggestions for better relational health:

Get counseling (if you are in desperate need)

Learn how to communicate effectively

Take a seminar

Listen more, talk less

Agree to disagree

Date your companion

Be spontaneous

Treat others as you wish to be treated

Love genuinely and completely

Suggestions for better financial health:

Get a financial advisor

Stop spending more than you have

Save more money sooner rather than later

Check your credit report and correct any problems

Begin to invest your money

Start your own business (network marketing or traditional)

Create a budget and stick to it

Spend cash instead of credit

Track your spending with free tools like Mint

Get your free credit score from Credit Karma

Suggestions for better physical health:

Hip Hop Abs

Tae Bo

Walk Away the Pounds

Turbo Jam

Fluidity

Yoga, Booty, Ballet

The Firm

30 minute power walking 3x's per week

Any activity that will get you moving and motivated to continue to change your life.

Proper Nutrition

Proper sleep schedule

Take a multivitamin

Cleanse your system of toxins

Drink plenty of water

Detox the body on a quarterly basis

Suggestions for better environmental health:

Buy healthier products that are environmentally safe Visit http://www.radiantlyyou.com/ahealthieru

Recycle and reuse

Be active in community environmental programs

Turn your home into a "Green" home

Teach your children about environmental health

Suggestions for better spiritual health:

Go to church, synagogue, temple, mosque etc.

Pray and /or meditate yourself

Pray with your family and/or others

Read the Bible or any other book that will strengthen your spirit.

Bibliography

Books

1. Grille, Robin. "Parenting for a Peaceful World".

2. Kyosaki, Robert. Rich Dad, Poor Dad.

3. Patchell-Evans, David, "No Sweat Fitness For The Rest of US."2005

Websites

1. Anisman-Reiner, Victoria. How can what you think and feel affect your health and the way you're living. (www.Natural medicine.suite101.com, June 10, 2006).

2. Davis, Sylvia. Boost Your Emotional Health WebMD Weight Loss Clinic. (www.medicinenet.com, 2007).

3. Kurtus, Ron. What is Physical Health? www.school-for-champions.com/health/whatis (Revised-22 September 2002).

4. www.self-renewal.com 2006.

5. Lerche Davis, Jeanie. Stressed Out? Chill Out, to Avoid Stroke, WebMD Medical News Aug. 2, 2001 (www.webmd.com).

Related Articles

Article 1

Complete article referenced in Chapter 2 Emotional Wellness –Boost Your Emotional Health

Experts offer 12 steps to emotional wellness.

By Sylvia Davis - WebMD Weight Loss Clinic - Feature Reviewed by Louise Chang, MD

* Collect Friends

* Enjoy Solitude

* Get Fit

* Seek Pleasure

* Find a Passion

* Plan for Problems

* Seek Constructive Criticism

* Take Healthy Risks

* Manage Success Well

* Don't Go It Alone

* Write It Down

* Protect Yourself from 'Energy Vampires'

You know you need to take care of your physical health, but have you been doing enough to maintain a healthy emotional balance? Here are 12 tips from the experts for reducing stress, managing negative emotions, and improving your emotional wellness.

1. Collect Friends

You need people, lots of them.

"If you look at all the theories of psychotherapy, people who have a lot of social support are happier," says Rebecca Curtis, PhD, a professor of psychology at Adelphi University in Garden City, N.Y., and director of research at the W.A. White Institute of Psychiatry, Psychology and psychoanalysis in New York City. The opposite is true, also. "We all need to be checking out our thoughts with other people, and people get weirder and weirder the more they stay alone," Curtis says. If the friends-of-friends-of-friends chain reaction that had kept your life stocked with new relationships has fizzled out -- for example, if you have moved to a new place where you don't know anyone -- try taking a more active role. But instead of trying to chat up folks at the local watering hole, sign up for a class that involves a lot of social interaction.

"It's easier to meet people if there's some kind of a structured discussion about a certain subject," says Muriel James, PhD, psychologist and author of Its Never Too Late to Be Happy.

2. Enjoy Solitude

This step may seem to contradict the first one, but actually it complements it. Some isolation can be quite healthy.

"The isolation that comes when people have given up on other people is the problem," Curtis says. Avoid this extreme, but don't be such a social butterfly that you lose yourself completely. Take time to "sit with your feelings," Curtis says, without distractions.

Some call this meditation, but it doesn't have to be done in the lotus position. For example, if you spend an hour alone in the car every day, keep the radio off, and listen to your thoughts instead.

Haven't got an hour alone? Try a three-minute meditation: close your door, turn off the phone, and then close your eyes. Take deep breaths, focusing on your breath as it goes in and out. If thoughts come to you, just bring yourself back to your breathing. Then think about a beautiful image, a flower, a child's face; look at every detail. Then, gradually, breathe faster and open your eyes.

3. Get Fit

We're not saying, "Look fabulous in time for swimsuit season." Just get your body moving. Study after study has shown that exercise lifts mood and generally enhances quality of life. I use the phrase go play instead of exercise because, it makes me feel less restricted if I think of exercise as something fun to do instead of cumbersome.

Break any vicious cycles you see happening, which get in the way of adding positive things like exercise to your daily routine. Booze, cigarettes, overeating, junk food, or all these combined are an impediment to physical activity, and overindulging leads to more of the same.

It's important for emotional health to maintain your physical health in all the ways you can. So get enough sleep; eat regular, balanced meals; and take time for relaxation as well.

4. Seek Pleasure

This may also seem like a contradiction, but moderation in all things is the message here. Everyone knows that "all work and no play makes Jack a dull boy." Overly rigorous devotion to work drives you batty.

Still, it's easy to become consumed by your responsibilities and to neglect your own enjoyment of life.

In his book, Your Own Worst Enemy: Breaking the Habit of Adult Underachievement, psychologist Kenneth Christian, PhD, directs readers to add something positive and pleasurable to their life, do it every day, and make it permanent.

5. Find a Passion

If you don't know what your purpose in life is, start smaller. "Make a list of things you want to do before you die," Christian says. Don't be shy about writing down wild schemes. If your first list is uninspiring, make another one. Keep making lists and look for any recurring themes.

Identifying an interest and pursuing it can develop into a rich and exciting life that you'd never imagined you'd have. "Not all that helps us reach goals is linear," Christian says. Ask yourself, "What cooks for me?" he says. Once you identify your passion, then you can put a plan of action in place to live out your passion every day of your life.

6. Plan for Problems

Instead of expecting everything in your life to go smoothly --
some things will, and some definitely won't -- or worrying about
what will happen to you if things go wrong, plan for potential
problems.

Some problems blindside us, but others are more predictable.
Muriel James gives an example: If you think you may have to
get up in the middle of the night, will you fret about possibly
tripping over things in the dark, or will you turn on a night light?

7. Seek Constructive Criticisms

"Often people are doing things to mess themselves up, but they
really don't have a clue of what is going wrong," Rebecca Curtis
says. For example, "They really may not be aware of how
they're acting with people."

You probably are very charming -- but maybe you are rubbing
people the wrong way. Too much self-consciousness can
paralyze you socially, but don't be oblivious to how others
perceive you.

The same goes for your work. Don't be afraid to ask, "Am I
doing a good job?"

8. Take Healthy Risks

People need to approach what they feel anxious about," Curtis
says. This doesn't mean you should force yourself into

terrifying situations needlessly. But if you never leave your comfort zone, your life will be all the poorer for it.

9. Manage Success Well

"If at First You Do Succeed, Try Thinking like a Woman," is the title of a chapter in Reclaiming the Fire: How Successful People Overcome Burnout, by Steven Berglas, PhD.

"Women hold on to relationships with competitors. Men litter the battlefield with corpses," says Berglas, a psychologist at the John E. Anderson School of Management at UCLA.

Spreading your success around, rather than jealously guarding it, promotes better emotional health by continuing to build your sense of self-worth. "If success ends your ability to build self-esteem, or if you're not building self-esteem, you're just resting on it, then you start committing crazy acts," Berglas says.

People who get bored with their success, he says, "start looking for ways to dare the devil and beat him." Eventually they lose.

10. Don't Go It Alone

Psychologists would urge just about everyone to get into therapy. None of us make it to adulthood emotionally unscathed, and there are mental health experts waiting to help you.

"It's the 21st century," Curtis says. "Don't be a dinosaur and insist on doing it all by yourself."

11. Write It Down

Identify negative thoughts and don't let them ambush you, says Judith Orloff, MD, assistant professor of clinical psychiatry at UCLA. "Don't beat yourself up for being stressed, but bring your fears into the open on paper. Make a list of your seven worst fears."

Then, she says, make a second list of the things you are grateful for.

Irwin says he did much the same with a family member who was getting down and negative. Parents need to teach children to make a list of positives, too.

Writing the negatives bleeds them of power. They become words on paper.

12. Protect Yourself from 'Energy Vampires'

The Drama Queen, the Sob Sister, the Constant Talker, and the Blamer – do you know any of these people? Chances are you do. And any of them can wear you out

You need to learn to set boundaries," Orloff says. "Listen for awhile, and then break off the interchange. People are so afraid to do this. They don't want to seem impolite. You need to be firm, though kind."

The same goes for technology, which can be an overwhelming stressor. "People go into despair when their computer breaks (or they forget their cell phone for a day).

"Don't let your computer hypnotize you. Get outside, at least look outside!"

SOURCES: WebMD Feature: "10 Steps to Emotional Health in 2005." WebMD Feature: "Spring Break Makeover for the Mind."

Article 2 - A Workout That Actually Works

Your 30-Minute, Tried-and-True Workout

You arrange your schedule and actually get to the gym, only to find yourself overwhelmed by the workout options there. Is it best to do cardio or strength? Machines or mats? You know the basic exercises, but you don't know how to fit it all together into a routine that works. Of course, a personal trainer could inspire and guide you, but at an average of $50 to $75 an hour, that's just not something everyone can afford.

What you need is a general workout that can help you stay toned and fit and is adaptable to even the tightest schedules—and we've got a great one for you right here! Here's an example of a 30-minute, all-around workout that combines cardio and strength.

The Cardio (15 minutes)

For this part of the workout, you're going to be focusing on the RPE or Rate of Perceived Exertion—this just means how intensely you feel you are exercising. Think of 1 as a slow walk in the park, when you're barely exerting any energy, and think of 10 as so much exertion it feels like you're going to pass out.

For the cardio exercises, you can pick any activity of your choice, like walking, jogging, biking, or using a treadmill or an elliptical machine.

- 3 minutes: RPE 4

- 2 minutes: RPE 6

- 1 minute: RPE 8

- 2 minutes: RPE 6

- 1 minute: RPE 8

- 2 minutes: RPE 6

- 1 minute: RPE 8

- 3 minutes: RPE 4

The Strength Training (15 minutes)

Complete two sets of 15 repetitions of the following 6 exercises:

- Bicep Curls

- Triceps Extensions

- Push-ups

- Shoulder Presses

- Lunges

- Squats

All in Your Time

This is great for those times when you've got a half hour, but the best thing about this workout routine is its adaptability. You can adjust it for those leisurely days when you want to extend your workout to an hour or for those days when you're so pressed for time that all you can afford is 15 minutes.

To adjust these exercises for more or less time, just increase or decrease the amount of time on each interval of cardio exercises, as well as the repetitions of strength exercises.

No matter who you are or what your level of fitness is, this is a general workout routine for you—one that can keep you energized and feeling your best.

Article 3

First Steps to Spiritual Growth: How to have meaningful time with God by Rick Warren

(Condensed from his book, Dynamic Bible Study Methods) Once you go about having one? You may be motivated to do it but may not know how. You need to consider four essentials elements of a good quiet time:

> Start with the proper attitudes.

> Select a specific time.

> Choose a special place.

> Follow a simple plan.

START WITH THE PROPER ATTITUDES

In God's eyes, why you do something is far more important than what you do.   On one occasion God told Samuel, "The Lord does not look at the things man looks at. Man looks at the outward appearance, but the Lord looks at the heart." (1 Samuel 16:7, NIV*) It is quite possible to do the right thing but with the wrong attitude.   This was Amaziah's problem, for he did what was right in the eyes of the Lord but not wholeheartedly. (2 Chronicles 25:2)   When you come to meet with God in the quiet time, you should have these proper attitudes:

1.   Expectancy - Come before God with anticipation and eagerness. Expect to have a good time of fellowship with Him and receive a blessing from your time together. That

was what David expected: "O God, You are my God, earnestly I seek you." (Psalm 63:1)

2.   Reverence - Don't rush into God's presence, but prepare your heart by being still before Him and letting the quietness clear away the thoughts of the world. Listen to the prophet Habakkuk: "The Lord is in His holy temple; let all the earth be silent before Him." (Habakkuk 2:20; see also Psalm 89:7) Coming into the presence of the Lord is not like going to a football game or some other form of entertainment.

3.   Alertness - Get wide-awake first. Remember that you are meeting with the Creator, the Maker of heaven and earth, and the Redeemer of men. Be thoroughly rested and alert. The best preparation for a quiet time in the morning begins the night before. Get to bed early so you will be in good shape to meet God in the morning; He deserves your full attention.

4.   Willingness to obey - This attitude is crucial: you don't come to your quiet time to choose what you will do or not do, but with the purpose of doing anything and everything that God wants you to do. Jesus said, "If anyone chooses to do God's will he will find out whether my teaching comes from God or whether I speak on my own." (John 7:17) So come to meet the Lord having already chosen to do His will no matter what.

SELECT A SPECIFIC TIME

The specific time has to do with when you should have your quiet time and how long it should be. The general rule is this: The best time is when you are at your best! Give God the best part of your day - when you are the freshest and most alert.

97

Don't try to serve God with your leftovers (leftover time).
Remember, too, that your best time may be different from
someone else's. For most of us, however, early in the morning
seems to be the best time. It was Jesus' own practice to rise early
to pray and meet with the Father: "Very early in the morning,
while it was still dark, Jesus got up, left the house, and went off
to a solitary place, where He prayed." (Mark 1:35)

Throughout church history many Christians who were used most
by God met with Him early in the morning. Hudson Taylor said,
"You don't tune up the instruments after the concert is over.
That's stupid. It's logical to tune them up before you start." The
great revival among British college students in the late 19th
century began those historic words: "Remember the Morning
Watch!" So we need to tune ourselves up at the start of each day
as we remember the Morning Watch. If Jesus is really in first
place in our lives, we ought to give Him the first part of our day.
We are to seek His Kingdom first (see Matthew 6:33). Doctors
tell us that the most important meal of the day is breakfast. It
often determines our energy levels, alertness, and even moods
for the day. Likewise, we need a "spiritual breakfast" to start our
day off right.

Finally, in the morning our minds are uncluttered from the day's
activities. Our thoughts are fresh, we're rested; tensions have not
yet come on us, and it's usually the quietest time. One mother
sets her alarm clock for 4 a.m., has her quiet time, goes back to
bed, and then rises when everyone else in the household gets up.
Her explanation is that with kids around the house all day, early
morning is the only time when it is quiet and she can be alone
with God. It works for her; you need to select a time that will

work for you. You might even consider having two quiet times (morning and night). Dawson Trotman, founder of the

Navigators, used to have code letters for his night quiet time: HWLW. Whenever he was with a group of people at night or home with his wife and the conversation seemed to be ending, he would say, "All right, HWLW." HWLW stood for "His Word the Last Word;" and he practiced that through the years as a way of ending a day with one's thoughts fixed on the Lord (Betty Lee Skinner, Daws, Zondervan, 1974, p. 103). Stephen Olford, a great Christian and minister in New York for many years, said, "I want to hear the voice of God before I hear anyone else's in the morning, and His is the last voice I want to hear at night." David and Daniel even met with the Lord three times each day (see Psalm 55:17; Daniel 6:10).

Whatever time you set, be consistent in it. Schedule it on your calendar; make an appointment with God as you would with anyone else. Make a date with Jesus! Then look forward to it and don't stand Him up. A stood-up date is not a pleasant experience for us, and Jesus does not like to be stood up either. So make a date with Him and keep it at all costs. The question is often asked, "How much time should I spend with the Lord?" If you've never had a consistent quiet time before, you may want to start with seven minutes (Robert D. Foster, Seven Minutes with God, NavPress, 1997) and let it grow naturally. You should aim to eventually spend not less than 15 minutes a day with the Lord. Out of 168 hours we all have during a given week, 1 hour and 45 minutes seems terribly small when you consider that you were created to have fellowship with God. Here are some additional guidelines:

Don't try for a two-hour quiet time at first. You'll   only get discouraged. You must grow in this   relationship as you do in any other. So begin with a consistent seven minutes and let it grow; it's better to be consistent with a short time than to meet for an hour every other week.

Don't watch the clock. Clock-watching can ruin your quiet time faster than almost anything else. Decide   what you can do in the Word and prayer during the   time you have selected; then do it. Sometimes it will take longer than you have set aside and sometimes less time. But don't keep looking at your watch.

Don't emphasize on quantity, emphasize on quality. There is nothing super spiritual about have a two-hour   quiet time. It's what you do during your time - 15 minutes or two hours or anything in between - that's important. Aim for a quality relationship with the Lord.

CHOOSE A SPECIAL PLACE

The location where you have your quiet time is also important. The Bible indicates that Abraham had a regular place where he met with God (Genesis 19:27). Jesus had a custom of praying in the Garden of Gethsemane on the Mount of Olives. "Jesus went out as usual to the Mount of Olives, and His disciples followed Him." (Luke 22:39, emphasis added)   Your place ought to be a secluded place. This is a place where you can be alone, where it's quiet, and where you will not be disturbed or interrupted. In today's noisy Western World, this may take some ingenuity, but it is necessary. It ought to be a place where you can pray aloud without disturbing others; where you have good lighting for reading (a desk, perhaps); where you are comfortable. (WARNING: Do not have your quiet time in bed. That's too comfortable!) .Your place ought to be a special place. Wherever you decide to meet with the Lord, make it a special place for you and Him. As the days go by, that place will come to mean a lot to you because of the wonderful times you have there with Jesus Christ. Your place ought to be a sacred place. This is where you meet with the living God. Where you meet the Lord can be just as holy as the place where Abraham met God. You don't have to be in a church building. People have had their quiet times in their cars parked in a quiet place, in an empty closet at home, in their backyards, and even in a baseball dugout. Each of these places has become sacred to them.

FOLLOW A SIMPLE PLAN

Someone has said, "If you aim at nothing, you are sure to hit it!" To have a meaningful quiet time, you will need a plan or some kind of general outline to follow. The main rule is this: Keep your plan simple. You will need the following three items for your planned quiet times:

A Bible - a contemporary translation (not a paraphrase) with good print, preferably without notes.

A notebook for writing down what the Lord shows you, and for making a prayer list.

A hymnbook - sometimes you may want to sing in your praise time (see Colossians 3:16).

1. Wait on God (Relax). Be still for a minute; don't come running into God's presence and start talking immediately. Follow God's admonition: "Be still and know that I am God." (Psalm 46:10; see also Isaiah 30:15; 40:31) Be quiet for a short while to put yourself into a reverent mood.

2. Pray briefly (Request). This is not your prayer time, but a short opening prayer to ask God to cleanse your heart and guide you into the time together.

Two good passages of Scripture to memorize are:

"Search me, O God, and know my heart; test me and know my anxious thoughts. See if there is any offensive way in me, and lead me in the way everlasting." (Psalm 139:23-24; see also 1 John 1:9)

Open my eyes that I may see wonderful things in your law [the Word]." (Psalm 119:18; see also John 16:13) You need to be in tune with the Author before you can understand His Book!

3. Read a section of the Scripture (Read). This is where your conversation with God begins. He speaks to you through His Word, and you speak with Him in prayer. Read your Bible slowly. Done Repeatedly. Read a passage over and over until you start to picture it in your mind. The reason more people don't get more out of their Bible reading is that they do not read the Scriptures repeatedly. Without stopping. Don't stop in the middle of a sentence to go off on a tangent and do a doctrinal study. Just read that section for the pure joy of it, allowing God to speak to you. Remember that your goal here is not to gain

information, but to feed on the Word and get to know Christ better. Aloud but quietly. Reading it aloud will improve your concentration, if you have that problem. It will also help you understand what you are reading better because you will be both seeing and hearing what you are reading. Read softly enough, however, so that you won't disturb anyone.

Systematically. Read through a book at a time in an orderly method. Do not use the "random dip" method - a passage here, a chapter there, what you like here, an interesting portion there. You'll understand the Bible better if you read it as it was written - a book or letter at a time. To get a sweep of a book. On some occasions you may want to survey a whole book. In that case you will read it quickly to get a sweep of the total revelation. Then you need not read it slowly or repeatedly.

4. Meditate and memorize (Reflect and Remember). In order to have the Scriptures speak to you meaningfully, you should meditate on what you are reading and memorize verses that particularly speak to you. Meditation is "seriously contemplating a thought over and over in your mind." Out of your meditation you might select and memorize a verse that is particularly meaningful to you.

5. Write down what God has shown you (Record). When God speaks to you through His Word, record what you have discovered. Writing it down will enable you both to remember what God revealed to you and to check up on your biblical discoveries. Recording what God has shown

you is the way of applying what you see in the Scripture that pertains to your life.

6. Have your time of prayer (Request). After God has spoken to you through His Word, speak to Him in prayer. This is your part of the conversation with the Lord.

CONCLUSION

What if you miss a day? Don't worry about it if it only happens occasionally. Don't go on a guilt trip. "There is now no condemnation for those who are in Christ Jesus. (Romans 8:1, NIV)   Don't get legalistic because missing one day does not make it a flop. BUT don't give up. If you miss a meal, it does not mean that you should give up eating because you're inconsistent. You simply eat a little more at the next meal and go on from there. This same principle is true with your quiet time.   Psychologists tell us that it usually takes three weeks to get familiar with some new task or habit; it takes another three weeks before it becomes a habit. The reason why many people are not successful in their quiet times is because they have never made it past that six-week barrier. For your quiet time to become a habit, you must have had one daily for at least six weeks.   William James had a famous formula for developing a habit (Selected Papers on Philosophy, E. P. Dutton & Co., 2000, pp. 60-62):

1. Make a strong resolution (vow). You must always start with a strong initiative. If you begin halfheartedly, you'll never make it. Make a public declaration by telling others about your decision.

2. Never allow an exception to occur until the new habit is securely rooted in your life. A habit is like a ball of twine. Every time you drop it, many strands are unwound. So never allow the "just this once" to occur. The act of yielding weakens the will and strengthens the lack of self-control.

3. Seize every opportunity and inclination to practice your new habit. Whenever you get the slightest urge to practice your new habit, do it right then. Don't wait, but use every opportunity to reinforce your habit. It does not hurt to overdo a new habit when you are first starting. To these suggestions I would add one more:

4. Rely on the power of God. When it is all said and done, you must realize that you are in a spiritual battle, and you can only succeed by the power of the Holy Spirit of God. So pray that God will strengthen you and depend on Him to help you develop this habit for His glory. _____ If you have been convinced that this is what you need to do, would you pray the following:

A PRAYER OF COMMITMENT

"Lord I commit myself to spending a definite time with you every day, no matter what the cost. I am depending on your strength to help me to be consistent." This article was adapted from Dynamic Bible Study Methods (Chariot Victor Books, 1989) by Rick Warren. *All scripture references from the New International Version.

You may use this study guide for yourself or share it with friends, but please keep the copyright information within the document, and please don't sell it.

Daily Affirmations

Say these affirmations every day and you will notice a change in your thinking as well as a change in your life.

o   I am happy, healthy and whole.

o   I will have a gift driven life.

o   I am a money magnet, I like money and money likes me.

o   I am abundant in every good way.

o   I love and approve of myself exactly as I am.

o   I am deeply fulfilled by all that I do.

o   I deserve the best and I accept the best, now.

o   I am open and receptive to all the good and abundance in the universe.

o   I know I am worthwhile. It is safe for me to succeed. Life loves me.

o   I am peaceful with all of my emotions. I love and approve of myself.

o   I breathe freely and fully, I am safe, I trust the process of life.

o   Money gives me choices and choices give me opportunities.

o   I will act as if it were impossible to fail.

o   I will own my own DESTINY.

o   I will protect my dreams at all cost.

o   I am whatever I choose and I will put myself in a constant state of joy.

o   I am competent in every area of my life.

o   I am creating my own DESTINY.

Quotations

"Begin to free yourself at once by doing all that is possible with the means you have, and as you proceed in this spirit the way will open for you to do more." Robert Collier

It's how you deal with failure that determines how you achieve success." David Feherty

"A champion is someone who gets up when he can't." Jack Dempsey

"First say to yourself what you would be; and then do what you have to do." Epictetus

"Go confidently in the direction of your dreams; live the life you've imagined" Henry David Thoreau

"The major reason for setting a goal is what it makes of you to accomplish it. What it makes of you will always be the far greater value than what you get." Jim Rohn

Appendix

Physical Wellness Assessment

The physical dimension involves encouraging regular activities that produce endurance, flexibility and strength.

Feel free to print this page and take the test.

Read each statement carefully and respond honestly by using the following scoring:

Almost always =	**2 points**
Sometimes/occasionally =	**1 point**
Very seldom =	**0 point**

_____ 1. I exercise aerobically (vigorous, continuous) for 20 to 30 minutes at least three times per week.

_____ 2. I eat fruits, vegetables, and whole grains every day.

_____ 3. I avoid tobacco products.

_____ 4. I wear a seat belt while riding in and driving a car.

_____ 5. I deliberately minimize my intake of cholesterol, dietary fats, and oils.

_____ 6. I avoid drinking alcoholic beverages or I consume no more than one drink per day.

_____ 7. I get an adequate amount of sleep.

_____ 8. I have adequate coping mechanisms for dealing with stress.

_____ 9. I maintain a regular schedule of immunizations, physical and dental checkups (including Pap smears and blood pressure and cholesterol checks), and monthly self-exams of breasts or testicles.

_____ 10. I maintain a reasonable weight, avoiding extremes of overweight and underweight.

_____ Total for Physical Wellness Dimension

Score: 15 to 20 Points - Excellent strength in this dimension.

Score: 9 to 14 Points - There is room for improvement. Look again at the items in which you scored 1 or 0. What changes can you make to improve your score?

Score: 0 to 8 Points - This dimension needs a lot of work. Look again at this dimension and challenge yourself to begin making small steps toward growth here. Re member: The goal is balanced wellness.

Spiritual Wellness Assessment

The spiritual dimension of wellness involves seeking meaning and purpose in one's life.

Feel free to print this page and take the test.

Read each statement carefully and respond honestly by using the following scoring:

Almost always =	**2 points**
Sometimes/occasionally =	**1 point**
Very seldom =	**0 points**

_____ 1. I feel comfortable and at ease with my spiritual life.

_____ 2. There is a direct relationship between my personal values and daily actions.

_____ 3. When I get depressed or frustrated by problems, my spiritual beliefs and values give me direction.

_____ 4. Prayer, meditation, and/or quiet personal reflection is/are important in my life.

_____ 5. Life is meaningful for me, and I feel a purpose in life.

_____ 6. I am able to speak comfortably about my personal values and beliefs.

_____ 7. I am consistently striving to grow spiritually and I see it as a lifelong process.

_____ 8. I am tolerant of and try to learn about others' beliefs and values.

_____ 9. I have a strong sense of hope and optimism in my life and use my thoughts and attitudes in life-affirming ways.

_____ 10. I appreciate the natural forces that exist in the universe.

_____ Total for Spiritual Wellness Dimension

Score: 15 to 20 Points - Excellent strength in this dimension.

Score: 9 to 14 Points - There is room for improvement. Look again at the items in which you scored 1 or 0. What changes can you make to improve your score?

Score: 0 to 8 Points - This dimension needs a lot of work. Look again at this dimension and challenge yourself to begin making small steps toward growth here. Remember: The goal is balanced wellness.

Emotional Wellness Assessment

The emotional dimension involves recognizing, accepting and taking responsibility for your feelings.

Feel free to print this page and take the test.

Read each statement carefully and respond honestly by using the following scoring:

Almost always =　　　　　　**2 points**
Sometimes/occasionally =　**1 point**
Very seldom =　　　　　　　**0 point**

_____ 1. I am able to develop and maintain close relationships.

_____ 2. I accept the responsibility for my actions.

_____ 3. I see challenges and change as opportunities for growth.

_____ 4. I feel I have considerable control over my life.

_____ 5. I am able to laugh at life and myself.

_____ 6. I feel good about myself.

_____ 7. I am able to appropriately cope with stress and tension and make time for leisure pursuits.

_____ 8. I am able to recognize my personal shortcomings and learn from my mistakes.

_____ 9. I am able to recognize and express my feelings.

_____ 10. I enjoy life.

_____ Total for Emotional Wellness Dimension

Score: 15 to 20 Points - Excellent strength in this dimension.

Score: 9 to 14 Points - There is room for improvement. Look again at the items in which you scored 1 or 0. What changes can you make to improve your score?

Score: 0 to 8 Points - This dimension needs a lot of work. Look again at this dimension and challenge yourself to begin making mall steps toward growth here. Remember: The goal is balanced wellness.

Environmental Wellness Assessment

The environmental dimension involves accepting the impact we have on our world and doing something about it.

Feel free to print this page and take the test.

Read each statement carefully and respond honestly by using the following scoring:

Almost always =   **2 points**

Sometimes/occasionally =   **1 point**

Very seldom =   **0 point**

_____ 1. I consciously conserve energy (electricity, heat, light, water, etc.) in my place of residence.

_____ 2. I practice recycling (glass, paper, plastic, etc.)

_____ 3. I am committed to cleaning up the environment (air, soil, water, etc.)

_____ 4. I consciously carpool; ride a bicycle, walk, etc. in order to conserve fuel energy and to lessen the pollution in the atmosphere.

_____ 5. I limit the use of fertilizers and chemicals when managing my yard/lawn/outdoor living space.

_____ 6. I do not use aerosol sprays.

_____ 7. I do not litter.

_____ 8. I volunteer my time for environmental conservation projects.

_____ 9. I purchase recycled items when possible, even if they cost more.

_____ 10. I feel very strongly about doing my part to preserve the environment.

_____ Total for Environmental Wellness Dimension

Score: 15 to 20 Points - Excellent strength in this dimension.

Score: 9 to 14 Points - There is room for improvement. Look again at the items in which you scored 1 or 0. What changes can you make to improve your score?

Score: 0 to 8 Points - This dimension needs a lot of work. Look again at this dimension and challenge yourself to begin making small steps toward growth here. Remember: The goal is balanced wellness.

Intellectual Wellness Assessment

The intellectual dimension involves embracing creativity and mental stimulation.

Feel free to print this page and take the test.

Read each statement carefully and respond honestly by using the following scoring:

Almost always =	**2 points**
Sometimes/occasionally =	**1 point**
Very seldom =	**0 points**

_____ 1. I am interested in learning new things.

_____ 2. I try to keep abreast of current affairs - locally, nationally, and internationally.

_____ 3. I enjoy attending special lectures, plays, musical performances, museums, galleries, and/or libraries.

_____ 4. I carefully select movies and television programs.

_____ 5. I enjoy creative and stimulating mental activities/ games.

_____ 6. I am happy with the amount and variety that I read.

_____ 7. I make an effort to improve my verbal and written skills.

_____ 8. A continuing education program is/will be important to me in my career.

_____ 9. I am able to analyze, synthesize, and see more than one side of an issue.

_____ 10. I enjoy engaging in intellectual discussions.

_____ Total for Intellectual Wellness Dimension

Score: 15 to 20 Points - Excellent strength in this dimension.

Score: 9 to 14 Points - There is room for

improvement. Look again at the items in which you scored 1 or 0. What changes can you make to improve your score?

Score: 0 to 8 Points - This dimension needs a lot of

work. Look again at this dimension and challenge yourself to begin making small steps toward growth here.

Remember: The goal is balanced wellness.

Financial Wellness Assessment

If you're looking to improve your financial fitness this year, it's important to first understand how you're already doing. The following will help you understand how you're doing financially, and where you can improve.

1. What percentage of your income do you save each month

a. 10 percent or more
b. Less than 10 percent
c. None

2. How often do you use a monthly budget to track and plan your spending?

a. Almost always
b. Sometimes
c. Never

3. When you make a purchase using a credit card, how quickly do you usually pay off the entire balance?

a. Immediately or before the end of the month

b. Between one and three months

c. I usually carry a balance from month to month

d. How many times during the last six months have you paid a bill late?

a. None

b. One to five

c. Six or more

e. Most of your major purchases are…

   a   …planned in advance, with money set aside to
          cover them

   b   …planned even though the funds aren't
always there to pay for them

   c   …unplanned or spontaneous

f. If you needed to come up with money quickly to pay for
   a major home repair or an emergency, what source would
   you use?

   a. Funds already on hand

   b. Funds from available
       credit

   c. No funds available
       without establishing
       credit

g. If you lost your job or main source of income, how long
   could you provide for your basic needs and meet your
   financial obligations?

   a. Three or more months

   b. One to two months

   c. Less than one month

h. The insurance I have to cover the loss of major assets including real estate, autos and personal property is…

    a. …enough to cover replacement costs

    b. …less than enough to cover replacement costs

    c. …unsure or don't have coverage

i. When was the last time you reviewed and adjusted your retirement plan?

    a. Within the last year

    b. In the last five years

    c. I don't have any savings for retirement

j. When you think about your ability to meet future financial obligations, you feel…

    a. …completely at ease

    b. …moderately concerned

    c. …very concerned

Give yourself five points for each time you answered "a," three points for each "b," and one point for each "c," then total your score. If you scored between 40 and 50, you're in great financial shape. If you scored between 20 and 39, you are off to a good start, but could still address some weaker areas. If you scored below 20, you need to rethink your financial plan, and make some big changes.

Regardless of how you scored, now is a great time to sit down and examine your financial situation. Write down your financial goals, and develop a plan of how to accomplish each one.

The above assessments are provided as a starting point for your wellness journey. Use them to help you define a plan of action as you move toward total wellness and life fulfillment.

Healthy Tips

Science has shown that having a TV or computer in your bedroom interferes with sleep. Even when they are turned off, they emit a negative sound and disrupt sleep and energy levels. Bedrooms should be a place of peaceful retreat to support quality sleep.

Learn to laugh. Laughter is a powerful medicine that helps us develop better perspectives during stressful situations.

A sound nutrition and exercise plan is among the most important factors in reducing stress levels.

The key to attaining better health is to develop a strategy to incorporate healthy decisions into daily life.

To reduce your current weight by one pound a week, you need to reduce your daily intake of calories by 500 per day 3,500 calories per week). An effective way to do this is to combine a reduction in calories with an increase in physical activity.

Being aware of how you want to feel in any activity makes it more likely that you will perform well and enjoy the activity, make it a positive experience.

Making positive lifestyle changes can add years to your life. One study of Harvard alumni found that those who stopped smoking lowered their mortality rate by 41%. Those who began a moderately vigorous exercise program lowered their mortality rate by 23%.

Science has now proven that people who are happier live longer than people who are not. Happy people also have fewer illnesses and make more money.

If you find it difficult to exercise for 30-minutes or more each day, just do five or ten minutes. Often you'll find it difficult to quit once you get started.

Listening to music can be a great stress reducer. One study showed that cardiology patients who listened to classical music for 30 minutes produced calming effects equivalent to a 10-mg dose of Valium.

Visualize with feeling everyday about the person you want to become. See yourself as being that person NOW. Your brain will take what you visualize and help you create it.

A power down hour will help ensure a good night's sleep. One hour before bedtime, prepare your body for rest. Spend 20 minutes doing light chores that must be done so you will sleep better (pack book bags, make lunches, do NOT do heavy cleaning), spend 20 minutes on personal hygiene and 20 minutes reading or meditating. If you only have 30 minutes, do each of these activities for 10 minutes.

Good Reasons to Exercise

1.　Increases your self-confidence and self- esteem
2.　Helps you sleep better
3.　Strengthens your immune system
4.　Gives you more energy
5.　Burns up extra calories
6.　Tones and firms your muscles
7.　Lifts your spirits
8.　Builds strength
9.　Improves endurance
10.　Improves your appetite for healthy food
11.　Increases your metabolic rate
12.　Strengthens the heart
13.　Helps prevent heart disease
14.　Improves blood flow to the body
15.　Improves efficiency in breathing
16.　Lowers risk of death from cancer
17.　Alleviates depression
18.　Invigorates the body and mind
19.　Reduces illness
20.　Helps you live longer

There are so many more reasons to exercise; this is just a starting point. Remember we were created to move, it's just that SIMPLE!

Resources

Suggested Readings:

Books

The Bible
Three Feet from Gold – Greg S. Reid
Dare To Dream, Work to Win - Tom Barrett
The One Minute Millionaire - Robert Allen
Success Principles - Jack Canfield
The Secret - Rhonda Byrne
Quantum Leap into Your Network Marketing Business by
Toni Coleman-Brown
Sacred Pampering Principles - Debrena Jackson Gandy
Rich Dad, Poor Dad – Robert Kiyosaki
You Can Heal Your Life – Louise Hay
The Fat Smash Diet- Dr. Ian Smith

Magazines

Women's/Men's Health Magazine
Fitness Magazine
Self
Real Life Real Faith Women Walking By Faith
Home Business Connection
Black Enterprises
Fortune Magazine
Charisma
Inc.
Body and Soul

Motivational Tapes/Videos (are a great resource for helping you change negative self-talk) YouTube is a great resource

If Caterpillars Can Fly, Then Why Can't I – Alvin Day
The Ultimate Edge - Anthony Robbins

Suggested Exercise Programs:

Turbo Jam
Slim in 6
Zumba
Core Rhythms
Hip Hop Abs
CIZE
Sweating In the Spirit
Walk Away the Pounds

Suggested Weight Loss Programs:

The Diet Free Life
Jenny Craig
Weight Watchers
The Fat Smash Diet
The 400 Calorie Diet

Network Marketing and Business Websites

<u>Network Marketing</u>

Youngevity

http://thewellnessarchitect.youngevityonline.com/

Total Life Changes

https://totallifechanges.com/ahealthieru

nSpire Network

http://ceeceemiller.nspirenetwork.com

<u>Cee Cee's Business Website</u>
Just Make Scents
Self-Care Nature Based Bath and Body
http://www.bit.ly/justscrubs

A Healthier U Lifestyle Company
Holistic Health and Wellness
http://www.bit.ly/ahealthieru

About the Author

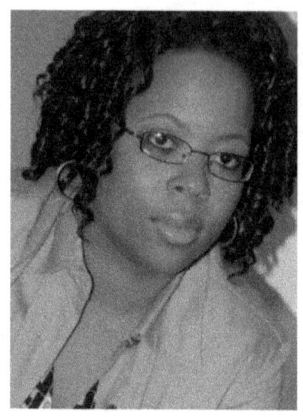

Cee Cee H. Caldwell-Miller, MA, CLC, ALS

Authentic Living Strategist, Self-Care Certified Consultant, Beauty Entrepreneur, Transformational Speaker, Information Consultant, International Best Selling Author, Performing Artist, Licensed Evangelist, and Certified Aromatherapist.

Cee Cee H. Caldwell- Miller is a native of Washington, DC and she now resides in Piscataway, New Jersey. Cee Cee attended Trenton State College in Ewing Township, New Jersey where she received a B.A. in Communication with a minor in African American Studies. She worked in the following industries: real estate, healthcare, retail, banking, higher education and software before deciding to pursue her Master's degree. Her love for helping people, since she was young prompted her to pursue a M.A. in Counseling, Human Services and Guidance with a Substance Awareness Coordinator, Cert. of Eligibility. She believes in continual education no matter what because applied knowledge is potential power.

Cee Cee has had a love for writing since she was 5 years old when her mother use to tell her to go write a story to get rid of her. Cee Cee began writing poetry, then she moved to writing one act plays, then into article/blog writing and finally to book writing. She believes that everyone has a story to tell. Her love for the written and spoken word has increased as the years have gone by. In 2008, Cee Cee released the 1st edition of her 1st book titled *Be in Good Health: Living a Life of Happiness, Wholeness and Wellness* which endeavors to help people live their best life, from the inside out in the 8 dimensions of wellness. Cee Cee released *Unspoken Words "Love" Vol. I* in October 2014 and has co-authored *Network to Increase Your Net Worth* in 2013 and *Tainted Elegance* in 2014, and varies other anthologies.

In 2015, Cee Cee was signed to Imani Faith Publishing and released *Stewardship and Service: God's Way or Our Way* in Spring 2016. She is also a part of *No Test No Testimony*, which is an anthology written to encourage people that they can make it through whatever they may be experiencing in their lives. She also became Senior Managing Editor of *Real Life Real Faith Women Walking by Faith Magazine* in 2015, which she knows will change women's lives for the better.

Cee Cee speaks and facilitates workshops on the following topics: **Being a Healthier U (Living Your Best Life From**

The Inside Out), The ABC's of Business Basics, Success Principles, Passion and Purpose, Authentic Living, Wellness In The Workplace, The Art of Relaxing, Relating and Releasing, Kingdom Stewardship and Servant Leadership just to name a few. She has helped many people on their journey to reach and attain BUSINESS & PERSONAL SUCCESS and WELLNESS in their lives.

Cee Cee is a member of Sigma Gamma Rho Sorority, Inc., Real Sisters Rising Women Business Association, the Womens Speakers Association and other organizations and groups. Cee Cee through her writing is here to help you reconnect with your passion, rediscover your strengths, regain your confidence, fulfill your purpose and gain life fulfillment and personal achievement authentically.

Cee Cee currently resides in Piscataway, New Jersey with her husband J. T. Miller. Her favorite scripture is "I can do ALL things through Christ who strengthens me!"Cee Cee believes that "You must READ to SUCCEED, because Readers are Leaders!" Through her speaking, workshops and books she hopes to **Encourage, Enlighten and Empower** *others to walk in their* **GREATNESS** *by living an* **AUTHENTIC AND INTENTIONAL LIFE ON PURPOSE!**

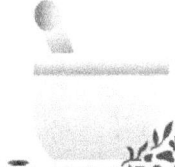

The Wellness Architect

RENOVATE, REBUILD, REVIVE.......

Your Mind, Your Body and Your Soul!

Cee Cee H. Caldwell-Miller AKA "The Wellness Architect" is available for hosting, coaching, speaking engagements, media appearances, workshops, pampering sessions, seminars or trainings by contacting her below at:

A Healthier U Lifestyle Co. (a division of)
Brilliance in U International, LLC.
Phone: (732) 497-2610)
http://www.bit.ly/ahealthyu

http://www.bit.ly/bewelltoday

beahealthieru@aol.com

To order additional copies of
"Be In Good Health"
Send email to – beahealthieru@aol.com
Cee Cee Wellness Library
http://www.bit.ly/wellnesslibrary

Other Titles Include:
EBooks/Books - (soon to be released)

Unspoken Words – Love, Life and Pain Volumes 2 - 4
The ABC's of Business Basics
The ABC's of Aromatherapy and Essential Oils
The ABC's of Self-Care

Blogs

The Wellness Zone
http://www.beahealthieru.worpress.com

Social Media Sites

Facebook

https://www.facebook.com/ladyceeceemiller

https://www.facebook.com/thewellnessarchitect

Twitter

http://www.twitter.com/beahealthyu

Pinterest

http://www.pinterest.com/ahealthieru/

LinkedIn

http://www.linkedin.com/in/ceeceecaldwellmiller/

Instagram

http://instagram.com/ladyceeceemiller

WELLNESS NOTES